FROM ANAPHYLAXIS TO BUTTERCREAM

THE AMAZING STORY OF HOW ONE MOTHER HELPED HER DAUGHTER WORK THROUGH LIFE-THREATENING FOOD ALLERGIES

Holli Bassin, MBA, Health Coach

ACCEDE CORPORATION PUBLISHING

Boston, Massachusetts

www.yourfoodallergycoach.com, www.hollibassin.com

Cover photography and design by KasZucker Design and Marketing.
Cover image courtesy of Treat Cupcake Bar.
Interior design by Amanda Filippelli.
Edited by Melissa Caminneci.

Hardcover ISBN 978-0-9985630-2-2
Paperback ISBN 978-0-9985630-0-8
E-Book ISBN 978-0-9985630-1-5
Library of Congress Control Number 2017930484

Printed in the United States of America.

A Note to the Reader

Acknowledgments

I'd like express my love and gratitude to my daughter, Rachel for her intelligence, perseverance, nonchalance and ability to think outside the box. I'd also like to thank my daughter Iris for her never ending smile and ability to always see the positive in anything and everything we ever do.

Loving thanks to my husband, Ed for his unyielding emotional support and enthusiasm throughout this process. His reasoning, intellectual perspective and positive outlook will always keep me buoyant!

Most of all I want to express my utmost respect and gratitude to Alexis. Without her knowledge, experience, dedication, perseverance, love and guidance we would not be living a normal allergy-free life today.

Honorable appreciation goes to the School of Integrative Nutrition for enlightening me about nutrition, immune system health, and coaching. This education has changed my and my family's life for the better in so many ways.

Exceptional thanks to my editor, Melissa Caminneci for her amazing hard work, professionalism, dedication, expertise, and guidance. I give her kudos for willing to work with me as a first time author and taking lead of the overall process.

Gratitude and special appreciation to Wendie Trubow for her expertise and leadership. And extraordinary thanks to Jenny Berk for her mentorship and passion for life!

Others to thank...

Scott Buquor, Deborah Elbaum, Nicole Crossman, Joseph Lipchitz, Jillian Erdos, Jean Sharry, Elizabeth Lee, Cissie Klavens, Debra Bruckner, Lena Goodwin, Holly Palli, Robin Zucker, Melissa Patz, Rebecca Young, and Sharon Goodfriend.

Contents

In loving memory of my Grandmother Miriam, my mentor and inspiration.

Goblin Free Treats

OCTOBER 31, 2015
It's Halloween and my two girls, Rachel, 12 and Iris, 10 are going trick or treating with respective friends. Two things are unusual about this particular event. First, Rachel is free to be at a neighbor's house for dinner and subsequently with her friends for the rest of the evening without any dietary restrictions, and second Rachel is actually allowed to eat *milk chocolate* anytime she wants.

Three years ago, Rachel would have had an allergic reaction to anything that contained eggs, dairy, or mustard. If she had ingested even a morsel of any of these foods, she could have gone into a life threatening state of anaphylactic shock, a severe allergic reaction. Initially after ingestion, she might have had a runny nose or skin rash. But within 30 minutes or so, she would have begun to feel nausea, tightness in her chest, itching, hives, swollen or red skin, tightness in her throat and trouble breathing. Without an immediate injection of epinephrine (adrenaline) to reduce the swelling she could have died.

Needless to say, I was always on guard and never more than 30 minutes away from her with an antihistamine and EpiPen in my purse, unless another adult was present who could administer the necessary protocol and call 911. In previous years, either my husband or I always went trick or treating with Rachel to be certain she didn't accidentally ingest anything that contained, or was made in a factory with eggs, dairy or mustard.

Some children who have only one or two food allergies can outgrow them. But children like Rachel who develop multiple food allergies rarely outgrow them. Rachel was only able to go from *anaphylaxis to buttercream* because I consistently analyzed and questioned the medical community's training and conventional wisdom of avoiding all allergens. As a result, we changed our mindset and opted for systematic desensitization, a non-conventional, holistic alternative method of allergy elimination that is managed with the guidance of a certified nutrition and health coach. In this therapy, once the immune system is balanced, the allergic client is given a precisely measured introduction of the allergenic food. The dosages are gradually increased until the food can safely be consumed without an allergic reaction. And it worked!

Here's Rachel's life changing story.

PART ONE
DISCOVERING FOOD ALLERGIES

CHAPTER 1

Our Bundle of Joy

Ed and I were married in the fall of 2001. Being on the mature side for a newly married couple, we wasted little time starting a family, and after nine months of marriage, I became pregnant. We were overjoyed when our healthy bouncing baby girl, Rachel was born on Red Sox opening day, 2003. We named our daughter after Ed's grandmother Rose, a Jewish tradition.

Though I was nauseous beginning at week seven of my pregnancy and the nausea didn't subside until sixteen weeks, I muddled through by eating crackers to help with the nausea. Otherwise, the pregnancy proceeded smoothly and I gained the appropriate weight.

At five months, I felt that first funny fluttery feeling-- a gentle kick from my unborn fetus. And at sixteen weeks I had an amniocentesis, a prenatal test to detect abnormalities that involved removing a small amount of fluid from the amniotic sac surrounding the fetus. The results reassured us that everything was fine. A huge sigh of relief!

THE "BIRTH"

At my 40-week appointment, the day before my due date, my OBGYN was concerned about decreased fetal movements. On that day, she did some tests in her office, but my kick counts were still too low, so she asked me to get an ultrasound. I picked up Ed, who was in a meeting with a client near the local hospital and together we went for the ultrasound.

During the ultrasound, the technician went into the adjacent office to call the doctor on the phone. The next thing I knew, my husband was on the phone with the doctor who was instructing him to take me straight into the Boston hospital for an induced delivery. Apparently the baby's amniotic fluids were at a dangerously low level.

My level of concern was less than that of the obstetrician. I had been participating in an online community with hundreds of other expectant mothers since the time of my conception. We formed our own support group and experienced each stage of our pregnancies together. There was a lot of information posted about pregnancies and subsequently deliveries where Pitocin, a synthetic oxygen used to induce labor was given for no reason except for the doctor's convenience, or to prevent liability issues. I was leery about having Pitocin. From my research, I knew that Pitocin made the contractions more painful and could result in an unnecessary cesarean section. I wanted my labor to come naturally and was convinced that our baby was not ready to come out.

Ed followed the doctor's instructions. But when we arrived at the hospital, I still refused the Pitocin. As I expected, the staff was unwilling to break my water because I was not in labor. Eventually I relented. They gave me the maximum dosage of Pitocin, but I still did not go into labor. Then they broke my water anyway. Despite all of the last-minute panic, my first labor and delivery was completely normal and natural, except for the epidural to alleviate pain.

Once she was in my arms, I enthusiastically began nursing my daughter in the delivery room. With the help of a lactation consultant my new baby girl latched on well. My milk however, did not come in for several days. I supplemented with Similac, and Rachel was voiding and stooling well.

CHAPTER 2

First Allergy Signs

The first sign that Rachel was in trouble happened when she was five months old. On a perfectly beautiful warm sunny day in September 2003, I seated my daughter in her Blue Evenflo stroller so we could go for a walk into town. At five months old she was sitting unsupported, an important developmental milestone; alongside her was a multi-colored huggable plush toy. In motherese I told her about the trees that had not yet started turning their brilliant New England fall colors. In response, she babbled away – "da, da, da, da."

Decked out in a short sleeve cotton pink and white striped onesie with a white bib decorated with whimsical flowers, a buzzing honey bee and the words, "Thank Heaven for Little Girls," with a pair of plastic kiddie sunglasses resting on the bridge of her nose, she was the living picture of the cutest thing ever! A beautiful, long, lean and curious baby, she had a twinkle in her hazel brown eyes and short baby peach fuzz hair that barely blew in the faint breeze. I loved being her mother and spending time with her.

Once we arrived in the town center, I stopped in the local ice cream store to buy a cup of black raspberry frozen yogurt. We crossed the street to the green park area so we could sit and enjoy the frozen treat. As Rachel had recently started eating solid foods, I didn't see any harm in giving her a little taste of the frozen yogurt.

Suddenly, her face and lips swelled and she developed hives. I had no idea what to do. I had never seen anything like this before. I panicked.

"Look at my baby!" I exclaimed to another mother in the park.

"Is this your first child?" she asked.

"Yes." I responded. She told me that she needed some Benadryl (antihistamine). I had very little idea of what Benadryl was. Luckily the local commercial pharmacy was right across the street and we rushed in.

"What should I do?" I asked the pharmacist in a trembling voice.

Calmly, he called the pediatrician's office to find out how much antihistamine to administer. I gave Rachel this dosage, purchased the bottle of liquid antihistamine and walked out of the store with my baby. Still shaking and numb, I didn't yet know that Benadryl would become as much a routine part of our lives as diapers, safety seats, Elmo, and Baby Einstein. While we walked home, Rachel fell asleep in the stroller, probably from the antihistamine. I felt baffled, traumatized, and scared.

The minute I walked in the door of my house, I called my husband who was on a business trip. Optimistic and not easily ruffled, Ed was his usual calm self. I was a wreck. He wasn't there to witness the experience. I told him it was like when the girl turned into a blue blimp in *Charlie and the Chocolate Factory!*

How could this be? What happened? Was it the black raspberries? It couldn't be the yogurt...or could it? At this point we just didn't know. And then, two months later we had another terrifying incident.

LAS VEGAS: NOVEMBER 2003

Rachel was 7 months old when the two of us accompanied my husband on a business trip to Las Vegas. Ed traveled often for business. He was the owner of a software company, and his clients were all over the country. This was our first time going together as a family.

While we were in Vegas, Rachel became fussy and began rubbing her body all over. Her skin turned a bright, blotchy red. Even her eyelids were red and puffy with eczema. As her eyelids were never swollen and red like that before, I knew she was having an allergic reaction. But to what? Then it hit me. Yogurt. I had been eating a lot of yogurt on the trip to try and combat what I thought was the start of a yeast infection.

What happens in Las Vegas, stays in Las Vegas, but all of this was not funny. I was still nursing and so she was ingesting whatever I ate. Ed was concerned about me because even though I was nursing, and it was hot in Vegas, I was drinking an excessive amount of water-- probably two gallons a day. So I began eating a lot of yogurt. Yogurt is fermented and contains probiotic gut flora to eat up the yeast.

What should I do? Clueless, I called the pediatrician. He told me to give her Benadryl. This relieved the immediate allergic reaction, but we wanted to understand the big picture.

CHANGE MY DIET?

Once we got home from Las Vegas, I asked Rachel's physician if I should change my diet. I suspected that Rachel may have been reacting to the yogurt, or more precisely to all milk products. The physician said it was unnecessary. Foolishly, I initially ignored my own instincts and listened to his advice. After all, doctors have years of education and training, so they should be knowledgeable and respected, right?

But a few days later, Rachel's eczema got so bad that I went ahead and changed my diet to see what would happen. I ate my cereal in the morning with either water or water mixed with a small amount of cow's milk as I wasn't aware of any other kind of milk at the time. Not very nutritious for me or for my breastfed baby, but just an experiment.

Lo and behold, in about three days I noticed a slight improvement in my daughter's eczema, something she had been suffering with since she was a newborn. Holy cow! She must be allergic to cow's milk! Should I change my own diet? What could I eat? Was she allergic to anything else? We just didn't know.

HYDRONEPHROSIS

Soon after Rachel was born, she was diagnosed with hydronephrosis or vesico-ureteral reflux. Hydronephrosis is a congenital condition of the urinary tract system that causes a swelling of a kidney due to a build-up of urine. Because of a blockage or obstruction, urine cannot drain out from the kidney to the bladder. The doctors put Rachel on prophylactic antibiotics to treat her condition.

All this rang a familiar bell. As a child, I had the same medical condition, which we were told was hereditary. My mother took me to some of the best New York urologists for treatments: Dr. Coleman and Dr. McGovern. I was constantly on Macrodantin, an antibiotic to prevent me from getting urinary tract infections, until at thirteen years old I finally outgrew the condition. I was told that I had high fevers as a child, and I was also on tetracycline which discolored my teeth. Subsequently, for years I had constant yeast infections.

And so, while I was always concerned about Rachel's eczema, at the time I was more concerned about the hydronephrosis and thought she might outgrow the eczema issues.

When I got back to Boston, I asked Rachel's pediatrician what to do. This doctor also told me not to change my diet. Though skeptical, I listened because I had no one else to go to who I trusted or from whom I could receive helpful advice.

Who could help me figure out what to do differently? I didn't know what questions to ask or why I should ask them. I did not know what foods were affecting our diet. It was very unclear.

I was fearful of giving Rachel anything new, but at the same time I was still in denial. "My daughter couldn't possibly be allergic to foods; that's silly." When I was growing up, children were occasionally allergic to nuts, but I had never seen an allergic reaction such as the one Rachel had experienced. I may have heard that someone got sick from eating a bad piece of shellfish, or someone may have had a peanut sensitivity, but literally turning pink with hives was completely foreign to me. I wanted to protect my daughter from ever having this happen again, yet at the same time I wanted her to live a normal life. And I was a new, inexperienced mother.

I begged the pediatrician to send us to an allergist for testing, but he thought it was unnecessary.

I was so confused and frustrated. I knew something wasn't right. Why did the doctor not see it? Finally, I chose to listen to my own intuition and eliminated all dairy products from my diet.

In the meantime, I began to wonder if the antibiotics that Rachel was on for the hydronephrosis might have something to do with her milk allergies that we first observed at five months and then at seven months old. Later I found out that they did indeed. They were killing the good flora in her gut, thereby weakening her immune system and natural defenses to foreign pathogens. Good gut flora is essential to kill bad, disease-causing bacteria in the gut and to keep us healthy. In fact 70% of our immune system is in our gut; our immune systems are dependent on good bacteria greatly outnumbering bad bacteria. But I didn't learn this until much later when I started to educate myself about the cause of Rachel's allergies.

Why didn't the doctors tell my mother to give me probiotics to replenish the good gut flora destroyed by the antibiotics? Likewise, why didn't the doctors tell me to give my baby probiotics along with antibiotics? Good question. Perhaps physicians are unaware of antibiotic's effect on the microbiome of the gut, or they know but ignore the implications. Whatever the reason, few bother to inform their patients upon dispensing antibiotics to also take probiotics or, if they do know, they don't emphasize the importance of doing so.

CHAPTER 3

First Food Allergy Signs

While Rachel had full blown allergy reactions at five months and then again at seven months, there were signs of potential allergies even earlier. At the time I was not educated to recognize these warning signs.

During our first pediatrician visit, when Rachel was four days old, the doctor discussed thrush with me as Rachel had some "baby acne." Thrush and yeast are related, but at this time I had no idea what was to come and so I didn't see this as a red flag. With the need to increase my milk supply, exhaustion from too little sleep, and Rachel's hydronephrosis, I had enough to worry about.

When Rachel was four or five weeks old, she had a rash on her chest and crusty ears. The pediatrician put her on Amoxicillin, an antibiotic. Around this time, we took a six-week Baby and Me class at Great Beginnings in Brookline, Massachusetts. During our very first class, the instructor pointed out that Rachel had eczema on her face. This instructor was also a registered nurse, lactation consultant, and mother/baby nurse educator.

We had also recently noticed baby acne on our daughter's face, but it seemed to be clearing up on its own and I didn't feel concerned. After all, I assumed the pediatrician was on top of it. Little did I know that that "baby acne" was a sign of food allergies that would soon consume our family's life and put my baby's life at peril, something the doctors had missed.

Still, the question of why she had a rash on her chest at all nagged at me. Why would there be an issue with her immune system? After all, I was breast feeding; I assumed she was getting all of the immunity and antibodies she needed from my milk.

INCREASING ECZEMA: SEPTEMBER 2003
By the time Rachel was 5 months old, I started to have real concerns about the eczema, which was getting worse. At this time, she also started to commando crawl. As she started crawling, she would rub her little itchy, rosy-cheeked face on the rug to scratch it. The eczema on her body got so bad that my husband started nicknaming her "little bunches of O's and P's with eczema behind her knees."

SOLID FOODS
It was also at around 5 months of age that we started introducing solid baby foods such as squash and rice

cereal. We were advised by our pediatrician to try one food for a few days before we tried the next. This would isolate any possible incidents or allergic reactions as had happened with the tiny bit of yogurt. We were still nursing and I had no idea what "safe foods" were or what she or I should or should not eat.

At six months of age, our precious daughter was now sitting up, giggling, and laughing. She was a happy baby and a joy to be with. She was mamma's girl. In fact, until this time I was the only one who could feed her because she refused to take a bottle. My husband used to call me "mommy milk cow," but at 5 months we started feeding her solid foods; baby cereal made with pumped breast milk which created constipation. Then we eventually graduated to store bought, jarred baby food including fruits and veggies. Apples and avocados seemed to be the only two foods she would suck on. My friend Karen had recommended that we try giving Rachel avocado, as avocados and breast milk had similar essential fatty acids. So I started buying the frozen pre-peeled avocadoes from Trader Joe's. This became one of her first "go-to" foods. For breakfast, she would eat carrots, rice cereal and avocado.

She also had trouble sleeping and a constant tummy ache; sometimes she would go three days without a bowel movement. But I had no idea why. As these were common problems in babies-- no one seemed concerned.

At six months, we tried working on sleep training. But Rachel didn't sleep through the night until she was nine months old. I would get up in the middle of the night, every night to nurse her. It was easy to just take her out of her crib and bring her in bed with me. That way everyone got a good night's sleep.

She also took the shortest naps in all creation! I used to call it the 42-minute nap.

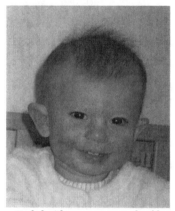

Rachel with eczema, 11 months old

And the eczema didn't go away. At this point, Ed and I suspected that the eczema indicated some type of allergy. But what allergens and what triggers? We didn't have a clue.

Ed had environmental allergies, so he suspected that her eczema could be from the chemicals in our laundry detergent or dust in the house. We changed our laundry detergent from Tide to a scent free, die free brand, but it didn't help. We suspected she might be allergic to the pink rug in her room. It had been left there by the previous owners, who had a dog. We considered ripping it out and polishing the hard wood underneath.

We were at a loss. Again, I begged the pediatrician to refer us to an allergist so we could find out what was causing the eczema, but he said there were waiting lists and she was too young for testing. Now what? Who could we turn to?

At 7 months she would eat a little baby cereal and about an ounce of green beans. At 9 months one of her favorite foods was raisins. I made a note in Rachel's baby book that "raisins were her favorite food, but she was allergic to grapes." The medical records also made mention of this at her 9 month checkup.

FEVER

Allergies are an immune system response. There were other signs that, in spite of the fact that I breastfed my daughter for ten months, her immune system was still functioning poorly. From the time Rachel was 10 months old until she was 11 months old (from Feb. 17, 2004 until March 18, 2004), her temperature ranged from normal to 102.9 for the entire month! I alternated giving her Tylenol and Advil with little effect. I couldn't figure out why this was happening.

And there was more. One day she was grabbing the left back of her neck, scratching a lot and eating poorly. I was beside myself.

Why would she be having a fever for so long? I asked the pediatrician to do a urinalysis but he refused. I asked again, but he still refused even though the urologist recommended one every couple of months. He didn't think she could have a urinary tract infection because she was on a prophylactic antibiotic, and he didn't want to do a culture because he said he had never seen a breakthrough infection while a patient was on prophylactic antibiotics.

The pediatrician thought the fever was probably just a virus even though she had no fluid in her nose, throat, ears, or chest. He condescendingly asked discouraging questions like "Are you first time parents?"

I considered calling the urologist to have him intervene, but I second guessed myself. Perhaps I was overreacting and he really did know what he was doing.

Finally, I showed him my notebook which documented her month-long fever. At last, he did a urinalysis.

When he called to tell me the results of the culture, he had an undertone of embarrassment or uncertainty in his voice. Something was not right, but he didn't elaborate. He simply gave instructions for a new antibiotic without explanation.

The urine culture showed e-coli in her urinary tract that was resistant to amoxicillin. He changed her antibiotic prescription to Bactrim. That morning, my baby

FROM ANAPHYLAXIS TO BUTTERCREAM

took a three- hour nap. Her little body was exhausted from trying to fight the infection.

I was furious with the pediatrician. I felt disrespected and betrayed. A doctor needs to be a partner with his patient's care. He never asked us if Rachel had other symptoms such as foul smelling urine. The fact that I was a first time parent had nothing to do with my daughter's month-long fever or his failure to order a urinalysis, against the urologist's orders.

It was time to find a new pediatrician. I wrote a letter to the pediatric department requesting a copy of her entire file be sent to me as soon as possible.

We carefully selected our new pediatrician by talking with other parents and met with her the next month. Fortunately, she was enthusiastic and positive!

FIRST ALLERGIST APPOINTMENT: MARCH 2004

Prior to Rachel's E-coli infection, I finally convinced the first pediatrician to refer us to an allergist and we met with her shortly before our daughter's first birthday. She did skin testing on Rachel's back instead of her arms so she wouldn't be able to scratch the little bumps once the testing results showed positive for a particular allergen.

RESULTS

Soon after we got home, we received a call from the doctor with the results. Rachel tested positive for milk

• 23 •

– no surprise there! -- casein (the major protein in milk, the other being whey), egg white, egg yolk, oatmeal, almond, salmon, mixed shellfish, chicken, turkey, and grape.

Finally, answers! What a relief. The allergist gave us a treatment plan to follow. No more stabs in the dark. We now knew what we had to do.

To start, Rachel had to of course avoid milk, egg, chicken, raspberry, grape, almond, oat, salmon, turkey, shellfish (lobster, shrimp, crab) both in her diet and in mine, as I was still nursing. This was different than what the pediatrician instructed. He told me to continue eating everything, but now that we had the results of the skin test, the rules were changing.

At the first sign of an allergic reaction, we were to immediately give her Benadryl. If we saw any signs of a systemic allergic reaction - lip or throat swelling, choking, coughing, wheezing and or total body hives – we were instructed to go to the emergency room.

She was to get a bath daily and after the bath, we were to apply a moisturizer. If there was any sign of an inflamed rash, we were to use 2.5% hydrocortisone cream sparingly up to 2x/day, as needed. It also said to avoid dogs and cats.

RAST TEST
Subsequently the allergist ordered RAST Testing, a blood test to detect specific Immunoglobulin E or IgE

antibodies to determine what substances Rachel was allergic to. The RAST tested for allergies to cow's milk, casein, egg (white and yolk), soybean, peanut, wheat, oat, corn, rice, barley, beef, chicken, turkey, avocado, whey, latex, lobster, crab, shrimp, pistachio, lactalbumin, mango, and strawberry -- all common allergies. The test also checked for macadamia nuts, lanolin (wool), grape, salmon, raspberry, vinegar, onion, garlic, and lead allergies.

I was grateful that the allergist was so thorough in ordering the blood test as well as the skin testing, but I was also anxious for my baby. All of the physicians we had seen, including the urologist, pediatrician and allergist, wanted a set of blood tests from our toddler, a terrible thing for a baby to go through. Again, she would have to experience the pain and terror of having the needle stuck in her arm. Exactly one month after our first allergist appointment, I watched anxiously as the phlebotomist drew seven vials of blood from our one-year-old baby.

TEST RESULTS
The results of the RAST were overwhelming: Rachel had allergies to twelve different foods. What were we to feed our daughter?

We needed help! How could we feed our daughter AND reduce the reactions she was having while at the same time still provide her with the proper nutrition? Following the doctor's instructions to eliminate all of these foods from her diet sounded simple, but it was overwhelming.

Why was this happening? When would it stop? We were not given any explanation. We could only hope that she might outgrow these allergies and live a normal life.

VISIT TO ALLERGIST: AUGUST 2005
When our daughter was 21 months old, the allergist did more skin testing. She gave us a Treatment Plan and advised us not to give Rachel any peanuts or tree nuts. We were also told to continue to avoid milk/dairy, eggs, chicken, salmon, garlic, grape, and raspberry.

Each test gave different results that we found confusing. For instance, while the skin test results for peanuts were negative, the RAST Test results were (.66) positive, though Rachel had never eaten peanuts prior to testing. Almond was positive on the skin test, but that was not part of the RAST Test. Walnut was negative on the skin test, but she was never tested for it on the RAST test. Macadamia was not part of the skin test, but low (.11) on the RAST Test. She was never tested for pecan, cashew, hazelnut, or Brazil nut on either skin test. Pistachio was negative on the RAST Test.

The test also suggested an increase in her sensitivity to soy. Soy was now one more thing we started avoiding in her diet. Our babysitter, who came in a few hours per week so that I could work in my husband's office asked

"What am I supposed to feed her?" I wanted my reply to be "Welcome to my world!"

I prepared a list of some of her go-to foods:
- Chicken nuggets (always in the freezer).
- Ground meat:veal, lamb or beef (hamburgers without the bun were the only thing she could eat at a restaurant)
- Trader Joe's Fish Sticks: contained no eggs, whey or casein in the batter
- Crispix, Chex or other cereals, with strawberries
- Bagels, pasta, cinnamon Teddy Grahams, snap peas
- Cantaloupe, apple, raisins, and basically all fruits and veggies (as long as they were not cooked in butter)
- Mango and frozen avocado, both of which she loved.

At this appointment we were also given instructions to use saline nose spray 2x a day as needed for nasal congestion then blow nose and Dimetapp ½ tsp. up to 3x/ day as needed for allergy and congestion.

CHAPTER 4

Feeding Rachel

Now that we had testing results and were given the allergist's treatment plan, we had to learn to adjust to life while vigilantly avoiding the things Rachel was allergic to. Nothing could touch anything she was allergic to!

How does one live a normal life with food allergies? I was a nervous wreck. Sure I had control of what was purchased and what we gave her to eat, but what if inadvertently something in the kitchen contained an allergen? And I was completely uneducated as to reading labels. Fortunately, a nutritionist that the allergist recommended would meet with us in a few weeks.

Since I was still nursing, I also changed my own diet. I poured soy milk in my cereal in the morning instead of cow's milk. This is something that I had to get used to because I really didn't like it, but Rachel's health outweighed my taste buds. I consciously used only oil and vinegar on my salads. I ate soy ice cream for dessert. I bought soy yogurt, soy nut butter as soy was our new dairy substitute. I started reading labels more carefully, but I was still uneducated on all the ingredients that could contain the allergens that we were avoiding.

MORE ALLERGIES

So, all should have been fine. But it wasn't. Even with strict avoidance of the foods she was allergic to, Rachel still had allergic reactions and we had no idea why. One day she had a mild reaction on her face and neck. In trying to isolate what it could be, we thought it might be from the Puffins, a commercial breakfast cereal. We didn't know for sure. We were just speculating, so we stopped giving that to her. On another day, she had bad skin in the morning for no apparent reason. Her itchy eczema, a bright red rash that often appeared inflamed was often so bad that we sometimes gave her Benadryl before she went to bed for relief.

She was also still on prophylactic antibiotics for her bladder issues. Were they causing any of this? We had no idea.

Every new food became potentially suspect. We gave her fresh strawberries. Nothing happened. We gave them to her a second time and thought we saw a mild reaction. Even foods that were once safe might suddenly cause a new reaction. For instance, though she had been eating avocado successfully, on the morning of her first birthday we gave her some guacamole and *that* caused her to have an allergic reaction. Her entire body was red. She looked like she had a sunburn from head to toe. She was itchy and uncomfortable.

At home, at least I had control over her foods. But when we had to socialize, whether it was inviting guests into our own home, going to someone else's home, or being out and about, I lost control. As you can well imagine, this made me anxious.

RESTAURANTS

While a challenge, going to restaurants was manageable as we could bring baby food with us. We purchased plastic disposable high chair covers and placemats that I would keep in the diaper bag to protect Rachel from cross contamination in the restaurant.

PLAYTIME

Crawling everywhere though not yet walking, Rachel was meeting all her milestones and doing great. Miss social butterfly, she loved interacting with other infants. But for me her playing with other babies was a potential nightmare. Babies put everything in their mouths. What if she put something in her mouth that she might be allergic to? The thought terrified me.

We were already in more than one playgroup. How do you explain to others in the playgroup that you daughter cannot eat Cheerios? How do you stop your one-year-old child from accidentally picking up a cheddar goldfish from the floor from other crawling babies when your back is turned and popping it into her mouth?

I was horrified, and so were the other mothers in the playgroup. How do you impose the vigilance necessary to keep your baby safe on others without being a social outcast? It was hard. I tried to explain over and over to other parents how any item containing her allergens was potentially life threatening. But it was hard for other people to understand, and I felt very frustrated.

HAPPY BIRTHDAY RACHEL!

It was our daughter's first birthday. I was of course thrilled. We invited our friend Karen, her son, and a few other playgroup friends to join us, along with her grandparents from New Jersey. Rachel screamed with delight when she saw everyone.

She was growing up so fast. She was verbal from an early age, and we marveled at her utterings. If we said "A cat says meow," Rachel would say "ow." Grandma and grandpa were "gama" and "gapa."

All I could think about was how to make her cake. How do you celebrate a birthday without causing an allergic reaction? What ingredients could I use? My cake-decorating talents were limited to purchasing a cake mix, frosting, and disposable letter writing equipment from the supermarket and then doing a botch job decorating the cake. I had no idea where to find a decorated birthday cake without the ingredients Rachel was allergic to, and I was at a complete loss as to how to bake a cake using substitute ingredients.

What to do? Should I make one cake for her and another for everyone else? These thoughts obsessed me. Why? Rachel would have been happy with a cup of raisins. Perhaps because the cake thing was a reminder of how her first birthday was atypical. And I still had no clue as to why. Why was she so allergic?

I ended up buying a chocolate cake for our guests and wrote a note in her baby book, "None for you. You were allergic. I made a carrot and zucchini cake for you but you didn't like it." I could no longer deny the fact that my daughter couldn't eat birthday cake at her own party. I had to accept that this was not a normal situation and move on. It was so difficult to do so though when I couldn't explain why to myself, let alone our guests.

SIGNS OF HELP AT HAND

I needed help figuring all this out, so we hired Jenny, an MPH, RD/LDN and IBCLC Nutrition and Lactation Consultant to come to our house.

Jenny was recommended by the allergist and turned out to be a godsend. She had experience with food allergic families and was totally confident that she could help us. We needed someone to teach us how to read labels and determine what we *could* feed Rachel. Plus, since I was still nursing, I needed to know what I could eat. Jenny came to the door with professional attitude and her confidence and experience put us at ease. She brought with her valuable dietary and nutritional information for us to use as a reference.

HOLLI BASSIN

When Jenny arrived, Rachel was in the living room in Ed's lap. Immediately, she jumped onto the floor, stood up, held onto the long blue sectional and walked around us, staring at Jenny and babbling away.

Rachel was always inquisitive. As a baby, she had a furrowed brow that made you wonder what she was thinking. By 9 months old she started to communicate. Before she was physically capable of *saying* the words, we used "Signing Time" videos to teach her how to communicate via sign language. Very smart, she engaged easily in and mastered sign language for many words such as 'all done', more, cookie, juice, apple, cracker, milk, and water.

This was extremely helpful when feeding her because Rachel could sit in her high chair and let us know through sign language what she did and didn't want to eat. By the time she was a year old, her strong verbal skills -- she could say words like dog, bye bye, oh!, apple, OK, Elmo, (graham) cracker, up -- made it even easier to feed her. Considering her intuitive sense of knowing what could harm her, this was huge!

Jenny took out the information she had to discuss with us. She brought lists of foods that were considered common allergens, like peanuts, tree nuts, eggs, dairy, and more, foods that were usually hidden within packaging labels under different names. Today similar allergen avoidance lists can be found on the *Kids with Food Allergies* website, but back then this information was not yet available on the Internet. We were completely naive. We didn't know that there were other names for peanuts like artificial nuts, beer nuts, goobers, ground nuts, mandelonas, mixed nuts, and monkey nuts. We didn't know that casein and whey were dairy proteins, or that we needed to avoid certain brands that contained these ingredients, while other brands that were made in a nut free facility did not contain the ingredients that we were avoiding.

Some products said "natural flavors" and did not list the allergen. Also, there could have been a cross contact or cross contamination of the allergen with other foods. Different brands of the same foods had different ingredients: for example: Thomas' English muffins contain whey, a dairy protein or "milk" ingredient, while our local supermarket sold their own brand of English muffins that were dairy free.

Each brand had its own ingredient list. Jenny advised us to try other graham cracker brands because the one we had in our house was made in a facility with dairy ingredients, even though it didn't actually contain the dairy protein in its ingredient list. She told me to watch kosher labeling. For example - Ⓤ(D) stood for Orthodox Union made in a dairy facility and Ⓤ(DE) meant Orthodox Union made on dairy equipment. If something was strictly kosher it would be labeled as *pareve*, meaning no dairy would ever have the opportunity to touch that product. She warned us about cross contamination; even though a product did not actually contain the dairy protein, it could have contact with the protein in the facility if the facility was not completely dairy free.

We also had to learn about food families. For instance, since we were avoiding peanuts, she told us also to avoid sesame as they were from the same family. After this discussion, Jenny went through our pantry to teach us what we already had in the house that our daughter could and could not eat.

Jenny also taught me about *Oral Allergy Syndrome.* An allergy to birch may be associated with a reaction to other foods which cross reacts with pollen. These foods create the same allergic feeling in the mouth, but it's hard to explain to a child the difference. Also, while the raw food causes the oral allergy symptoms, many people find they can tolerate these same foods without symptoms when well-cooked.

So much to learn!

Jenny suggested we use a green sticker to label "OK" food. The list was getting shorter and shorter. And still we were at a loss as to why she had all these food allergies.

COOKING

The safest plan was to make our own food rather than rely on store bought meals. For instance, while store bought hummus often contains sesame, making our own would solve the problem. So we pan-fried tofu in oil, mashed it up with black beans or chickpeas, and used it as a dip blended with oil and spices. Voila! Homemade hummus.

NEW FOODS

Jenny advised us to try one new food every 4-7 days. We were to offer the new food plain, with no other new food. "Track it - try via a calendar so every "Monday" is a new food," she suggested. While we had to assiduously avoid any foods in any food families that Rachel was allergic to, it was safe to try: all fruits except raspberry and grape; all veggies; beef, lamb, pork; white fish; and all grains except oat. She advised me to eat Sunbutter (peanut/tree nut free) sunflower seed butter, IM Healthy brand.

As for drinks, she told us to give Rachel soy milk after weaning, approximately 20 ounces each day. She also suggested that we try Neocate junior (via prescription), which comes flavored or unflavored and to add the cherry vanilla flavor packet to it for taste.

INCREASING CALORIES

To ensure that Rachel was getting sufficient calories, Jenny told us to put oil on pasta, margarine on toast, bagel, English muffin, bean dip, gravy meatballs, to use milk free bread crumbs, pureed carrot, and milk free tomato sauce.

READING LABELS

Of course before we gave any food to Rachel we had to read the label, something we didn't know much about but had to learn as quickly as possible.

Labeling requirements now state that ingredients in foods must be listed by their "common or usual name" or the word "contains" must be followed by the name of the food source or (in parentheses). But in 2004, the FDA Food Allergen Labeling & Consumer Protection Act was not yet in effect on most products.

FAAN

Jenny also introduced us to Food Allergy Anaphylaxis Network, FAAN. This organization later became known as FARE, Food Allergy Research and Education. FAAN published educational materials about food allergies that my daughter loved, like *Alexander the Elephant* who was allergic to peanuts. Alexander was in many of the books we read to our daughter and became an important part of her bedtime routine.

COOKIES AND SOY MILK

I wanted to bake for Rachel so she could safely eat treats that all of her friends were eating, or at least were similar to them as food is an essential part of social interaction and of course cookies, cakes sweets equal love. Now, after meeting with the nutritionist, I learned how to bake using substitute ingredients for eggs and milk.

My first try at using Ener-G® egg replacer was an emotional roadblock. Honestly, I knew how to bake, but adding that extra step was a big hurdle. How was this powdery stuff made from tapioca starch and potato flour going to make an egg? I read the instructions on the box, measured the powder, and then warmed the already measured water in the microwave to make the "egg substitute" for the two eggs that it would replace in the cake. It worked. I made cupcakes with zucchini, carrot, soy milk, whole wheat flour, margarine (Fleischmann's non-dairy pareve) and Rachel loved them, screeching enthusiastically as she gobbled up the bite-sized pieces. She also started saying new words for the things she was eating like "pancake" and "cupcake," although she might not have been understandable to a first time bystander. I was excited because we could safely take the treats that I so lovingly made to a friend's house or the playground without worrying about her having an allergic reaction.

I bought *Dairy-Free, Egg-Free, Kid Pleasing Recipes & Tips*, a book by Theresa Kingma and started implementing some of her recipes into our daily life, including pizza and pancakes. I still have the book today and the Zucchini Bread recipe has a marker on it. This page looks very well loved!

Rachel would try anything I made, but she didn't always like it. The whole cooking and baking process was trial and error.

CHAPTER 5

Surgery & More Allergic Reactions

UROLOGY SURGERY: MAY 2004
At thirteen months of age, Rachel had bilateral re-implantation surgery at Children's Hospital in Boston. During this surgical procedure, the ureters (the tubes that connect the bladder and the kidneys) were removed from Rachel's bladder and reattached in a way that prevented the urine from backing up. This was new to me. When I had this condition, the urologists would cut and stretch my urethra in an outpatient procedure. Later on, urologists learned that the issue was further up the urinary tract. The procedure that Rachel had is now very common, and possibly the bread and butter of urology.

I was terrified that my now thirteen-month baby would have to go through a surgical procedure, as any parent would be. I was also anxious about her having anesthesia and sleeping overnight in a hospital. Of course I would sleep in the hospital room with her, but it was still horrifying to think about how well she would cope with the scary hospital procedure and the aftermath of pain.

I tried of course to do everything I could to ease the ordeal for her. I continued breastfeeding for extra comfort during and after the procedure. That wasn't hard as she was a fantastic nurser; though she was on solid foods, I still nursed her five times a day.

Rachel slept in the hospital crib with bars. She had an IV that we would carry along with us in the stroller as we walked her around in the hospital halls for exercise. When my friend Karen came to visit us in the hospital, she had to leave the room when the nurse emptied Rachel's catheter bag to give us and Rachel some privacy. It was awful!

After the surgery, a neighbor gave us *Madeline* by Ludwig Bemelmans. Madeline has appendix surgery in Paris--such an appropriate choice! It would be one of many favorite books and we would repeatedly read it to our daughter.

NOW ASTHMA
During Rachel's intake procedure in the hospital, we started talking with one of the residents. Food Allergies came up. "Food allergies, eczema, and asthma," he said, "are the holy trinity." She had not yet become asthmatic, but great! Now I would start worrying about this possibility.

This finally did happen in September of 2005, when Rachel was in preschool. She had episodes of 'coughing a lot' and the pediatrician put her on Pulmicort two times a day for asthma. She was too young for an inhaler, so, while watching TV she would inhale the Pulmicort twice a day through a nebulizer which was attached to a mask. We would call this her "fishy mask" time and she seemed to tolerate it. My little Rachel was such a trooper!

POST OP

Once we were home from the surgery, our troubles were not over. Our daughter was dehydrated and diagnosed with *C. diff*, a bacterium that can cause symptoms ranging from diarrhea to life-threatening inflammation of the colon. More antibiotics were necessary, including a strong prescription that we needed to fill from a compounding pharmacy because the regular local pharmacy didn't make it or have it in stock.

One night before bed, Ed gave Rachel the required measured dosage, but somehow he didn't inform me, so I also gave that dosage to her. It had a strong nasty medicine unlike the amoxicillin "pink stuff" that was so easily disguised with a tasteful flavoring. She then protested with a tantrum on the floor, almost as if she was saying, "Daddy already gave me my dosage." Of course, as she had to have the medicine and I was unaware Daddy had given it to her, I measured it in a syringe dropper and put it in the side of her mouth for her to swallow. When Ed and I later communicated and realized that we had each given her that night's bedtime dose, we felt awful.

ANTIBIOTICS AND MORE ANTIBIOTICS
Rachel had been on Amoxicillin, Bactrim and now a stronger compounded antibiotic. What were all these antibiotics doing to her immune system? Were they affecting her allergies in any way? In an infant who is beginning to develop her immune system, could the antibiotics have made the allergens worse?

These questions and the answers to them never emerged with the urologist, pediatrician or allergist as they were following normal procedure for a baby with hydronephrosis. Rachel needed to take prophylactic antibiotics to prevent her from getting a kidney infection and then to take Bactrim to resolve the e-coli infection, and finally the compounded antibiotic was needed to resolve the *C. diff* infection.

That all these antibiotics could be destroying the good as well as the bad bacteria in her gut was something of which they were unaware or considered unimportant. They never advised us to supplement with probiotics to reinstate the healthy bacteria needed for a strong immune system. Today, we now know how important this is. Almost weekly another research study gets published about how poor gut flora is the underlying cause of illness, from allergies to autoimmune disorders to even in some cases autism.

I trusted the professionals we were working with -- after all, they went to medical school and were experts in their field. Moreover antibiotics were supposed to be a medical miracle and safe. And so I blindly followed their procedure. Eventually I would learn better.

Fortunately, Rachel's urology surgery took care of the need for further prophylactic antibiotics as it permanently solved her structural hydronephrosis condition. We were thrilled! Now it was time to focus on living with food allergies.

NOT JUST FOOD

In the summer of 2004 we rented a house in North Carolina with my husband's immediate family. Rachel was 15 months old. I thought I had her allergies under control by restricting her diet. But then one day, when we took her swimming in the pool, she had an allergic reaction to the pool water. Hives and patches of eczema appeared all over her little body.

This terrified me. Now it wasn't just a matter of food restriction, there were also environmental triggers. These too would have to be investigated. Her little world was narrowing and it was profoundly disturbing.

RESTAURANT WOES

That wasn't the only troubling incident on our North Carolina family trip. We were still unskilled at managing food allergies in restaurants. One afternoon, we went to an outdoor buffet-style seafood restaurant with Uncle Stu, Aunt Audrey, and Cousin Emma. We checked with the restaurant manager for the ingredients in most of the items that we put on our daughter's plate, but apparently we didn't check the ingredients for the bread rolls and, as soon as Rachel put the roll in her mouth, she started developing hives all over her face and arms. We never found out what was in the rolls, but I assume it had either eggs, dairy, or both.

We dropped some cash on the table to cover our portion of the bill, hopped in the car with the diaper bag, which contained antihistamine, and drove back to the house.

Not all news was bad in North Carolina. On the last day of our vacation I told my husband I needed to go to the pharmacy to buy some diapers before we went home. I really went to purchase a pregnancy test.

To my delight and Ed's, the result was positive. At the same time we worried that the new baby could also have allergies and when I started nursing our new little daughter Iris, I was terribly nervous about what I should and should not eat. Luckily, she didn't develop food allergies like her sister.

ANTIBIOTICS VS. ALLERGY PREVALENCE
Whether or not I could have done anything to prevent Rachel from developing food allergies was more and more on my mind, as was the thought that the antibiotics for Rachel's hydronephrosis were the underlying culprit for her allergies.

But then I became unsure and confused after speaking with Madeline, an allergy coach colleague. Madeline had two daughters. Her younger daughter had hydronephrosis; she took prophylactic antibiotics but had no food allergies. Her older daughter did not have hydronephrosis and did not take prophylactic antibiotics but had multiple food allergies. What was going on here? One child took the antibiotics that I suspected might be at the heart of Rachel's food allergies and didn't develop food allergies, whereas the other daughter, who wasn't on antibiotics, did.

Was there a correlation between prophylactic antibiotics and food allergies, or at least a deficiency in immune systems, or wasn't there? Or could it be that Rachel's immune system never really had a chance to fully develop? Could medication for one condition affect another? How do doctors help the immune system recover from antibiotics? Questions, questions, questions!

Later on I discovered that cranberry extract and, even more powerful, the supplement D-Mannose flushes foreign particles from the urinary tract rendering antibiotics unnecessary -- something the doctors never mentioned! At the time though, I was at a loss.

BREASTMILK: NATURE'S PHARMACY
I loved breastfeeding, greatly enjoying the profound intimacy that my baby daughter and I had together. But after the surgery I was beginning to think about weaning. It would give me more freedom because I would

no longer have to worry about breastfeeding 3-5 times a day or bringing a breast pump with me to work.

On our vacation in North Carolina seemed a good time to start as Rachel was now 15 months old. So one day I tried to deny her a feeding. She started grabbing at my shirt; demanding to nurse. "I thought she was going to rip your shirt off!" my sister-in-law said.

As it turns out, my decision to delay weaning until after the surgery was wise. Breastmilk is nature's perfect food. But curiously, not all ingredients in breast milk are actual food for the baby. Breastmilk contains complex sugars called human milk oligosaccharides, or HMOs. HMO's are the third-most plentiful ingredient in human milk, after lactose and fats. But here's where it gets interesting. Babies cannot digest them. Why would this be? HMOs as it turns out are food for the microbes that live in the intestine, specifically one subspecies, *Bifidobacterium longum infantis*.

What this means gets a bit technical. So let me quote from a New Yorker article on the internet edited excerpting from *I Contain Multitudes: The Microbes Within Us and a Grander View of Life*, by Ed Yong.

"Human milk has evolved to nourish the microbe, and it, in turn, has evolved into a consummate HMO, a family of structurally diverse unconjugated glycans that are found in and unique to human breast milk. Unsurprisingly, it is often the dominant microbe in the guts of breast-fed infants... As it digests HMOs, it releases short-chain fatty acids, which feed an infant's gut cells. Through direct contact, B. *infantis* also encourages gut cells to make adhesive proteins that seal the gaps between them, keeping microbes out of the bloodstream, and anti-inflammatory molecules that calibrate the immune system."

In short, by breastfeeding, I was filling Rachel's gut with the bacteria it needed as protection from bad microbes and anti-inflammatory molecules. In other words, while the antibiotics were killing the good bacteria in Rachel's gut along with the bad, weakening her immune system and therefore setting the ground for her allergies, my breastmilk was brilliantly producing good bacteria to eat up the bad and reduce their impact. If I had not been a breastfeeding mom or had not breastfed for as long as I did because smart Rachel demanded it, she would likely have been a much sicker child than she was.

Of course I didn't know this at the time when I decided to start weaning which, as it turned out, actually started automatically with the new pregnancy–mother nature's plan exactly. Rachel rejected the colostrum I started producing for the new baby and was off the breast within a month.

Now if the breastmilk was boosting her immune system to reduce the bad effect on her microbiome from the antibiotics, then predictably she should have become more symptomatic when I ceased breastfeeding. And indeed this is what happened. Her eczema got worse. Of course at that time I didn't know why.

EPINEPHRINE INCIDENT #1

When Rachel was just under two years old, the allergist gave us a prescription for an EpiPen Jr, in case she had a life threatening allergic reaction and needed an immediate injection of epinephrine to save her life. Prior to that, our daughter's weight was below the recommended weight for this epinephrine product.

I felt relieved to have it but at the same time, I felt we had her allergies under control as the Benedryl seemed to do the trick quickly when she had an allergic reaction. Little did I know that we would shortly need this prescription medication.

On a hot summer day, when Rachel was two and Iris was about 5 months old, we all went to a volunteer parent-run non-profit organization Popsicle party at the Tot Lot a few blocks from our house. At the gathering were two boxes of popsicles. We carefully read the ingredients: one box contained plain non-allergenic popsicles, just high fructose corn syrup and water; the other box contained a milk ingredient (whey protein). We gave Rachel a popsicle from the allergy-free box, and I started chatting with some of the other parents. Shortly after, Ed ran up to me and started shaking my arm, "Look at Rachel!"

In just a few minutes, Rachel had hives all over her arms and torso. Ed put Rachel in the stroller, frantically ran home and gave her some antihistamine. It was a Sunday and the doctor's offices were closed, so I called our pediatric emergency line:

"How much Benadryl can I give a two year old?" I asked the doctor on line. He asked her state. "At this point, she's wheezing, no longer responding to our voices and barely breathing."

"Give her an EpiPen and call 911," the doctor responded.

My husband quickly grabbed the EpiPen Jr., read the instructions on the label, and jabbed it into her outer thigh, intramuscularly. "Ouch!" Rachel said. I sighed with relief. If she could say the word "ouch," it meant she was still breathing and still responding.

We called the ambulance. Ed went to the hospital with Rachel while I stayed home with Iris. When the ambulance drove away, I went outside to explain to the neighbors what had happened. "You mean Rachel is in that ambulance?" one of the neighbors exclaimed, hand on heart.

"Yes," I blurted, shaking all over.

The hospital was only about a mile from our house. By the time we called 911, waited for the emergency responders, and put her in the ambulance, we probably could have driven her to the hospital in a shorter time.

The reason this is relevant is because once Ed arrived at the hospital, it was hurry up and wait.

I originally stayed home with Iris, but ended up driving to the hospital with Rachel's two lovies, her stuffed Gund Elmo doll and "bebe," the cloth diaper that she slept with for comfort.

I brought Iris with me and the four of us hung around the hospital for four hours while the staff observed Rachel to make sure she would not have a second biphasic reaction. Rachel was delighted as she got to watch cartoon videos, something we tried not to let her do at home for too long or too often.

All this was emotionally traumatic. Rachel was fine once we got home, so we tried to act normal by going on with the rest of our afternoon and evening. But I was still a wreck. I wondered, why was this all happening and how could we prevent it from happening again? Someone might have accidentally put one Popsicle back in the wrong box, an innocent gesture, but it made the rest of our day crazy. The next day, I called the allergist and pediatrician, but there wasn't much they could do for me except tell me to avoid all dairy products. This was easier said than done.

CHAPTER 6

Normal Family Lifestyle Despite Food Allergies

SPRING 2005

I wanted Rachel's second birthday party to be special and to me that meant a sensational birthday cake. And I certainly did succeed. As a friend told me, she will never remember the party. "All you have to do is have a picture of the cake."

My friend Lori recommended a woman who owned a business called "Crazy Cakes." She made specially ordered personalized cakes from her home, and she turned out to be my cake-making savior. She agreed to bake an Elmo cake, without eggs, dairy, or nuts by using a Trader Joe's mix and a soy frosting (we were back to eating soy). I was thrilled because it would look professional and I wouldn't have to worry about trying to decorate it.

So, for Rachel's second birthday, we had a party in a rented play space in a school. We decided to combine the weekend with a baby naming for Iris, our new baby girl who was born around the time Rachel turned two. A lot of family came in from out of town, and we had a room full of people. We ordered an allergy-free deli meat platter to go with the cake for the event which turned out to be a success!

We still had to worry about allergies because we never knew if someone else would accidentally contribute to a cross-contact incident, but we were relieved that we had a family celebration without any emergency room visits.

THIRD BIRTHDAY: SPRING 2006

When my daughters were three and one respectively, we decided to have a combined birthday party. I contacted the same Crazy Cakes woman who was my savior the pre-vious year to bake a Dora the Explorer sheet cake with the same allergy-safe ingredients. Dora the Explorer was one of Rachel's favorite TV characters from the animated Nick Jr. show.

On a beautiful May sunny day, we had a party in the backyard with many different arts and crafts stations. The kids painted wooden boxes and made necklaces using pony beads and lanyards, swung energetically on the swing set in the backyard and of course devoured the cake!

The party was a big hit!

FOURTH BIRTHDAY: SPRING 2007

Prior to Rachel's fourth birthday party, I tried to get in touch with my cake making savior once again, but she was not returning my calls.

As I had no way to order an allergy-free cake, I signed up for a basic cake decorating class at our local AC Moore. Along with signing up for the class, I purchased a large pre-filled Wilton cake decorating caddy supply kit which included fifty of the basic necessary cake decorating pieces. I brought Rachel with me; she had a ball playing with the allergy-safe frosting!

CAKE CRAZY

After that, I started making cakes for both daughters' birthdays. After all, how could my older daughter go to my younger daughter's party and not be able to eat the cake? I used the castle cake pan multiple times with similar Disney themes. No two cakes were exactly the same.

SIXTH BIRTHDAY: SPRING 2009

For Rachel's 6th birthday, I used the same castle cake pan to make another princess cake. I found a company in Boston who rented out actresses and we hired an actress to come to our house and pretend to be Ariel from the Disney movie. "I really believe this is Ariel," said one mom.

I made a beautiful castle cake with all the appropriate colors and shimmery sprinkles all over. Since I was baking in my own kitchen with an allergen-free cake mix, egg re-placer and soy milk, we didn't have to worry much about cross-contact allergens. I was in control, but it probably took me the better part of five hours to bake, mix frosting colors, and decorate the cake. It felt heartbreaking to cut up the cake. Hours of work were gone in just minutes. But I was getting the hang of accommodating my daughter's food allergies.

Rachel and Iris and all the girls loved the cake! They were in princess fantasy land for the day, as was I. My mother, who visited from New Jersey, couldn't believe how much work I put into the cake. She too commented that it was a shame to cut it up.

This party was another big hit; we were on a birthday party roll.

When Rachel was invited to someone else's birthday party, I would bake an entire batch of cupcakes just so she could bring one allergy-free cupcake. I never could find any store-bought cake that she could eat. As Rachel made more friends and was invited to more gatherings, I learned to freeze the extra cupcakes for the next party. I was certainly getting the hang of this food allergy mom thing!

Every cloud has a silver lining and honestly, there is a bright side to all of this. We NEVER had eggs in the house simply because we didn't use them. I was used to baking and cooking with substitute ingredients, so when we had a snowstorm, we never had a reason to panic. While everyone else ran out to the supermarket to stock up on fresh eggs and milk, we were all set with our Ener-G egg replacer and soy milk which had a longer shelf life.

VACATIONS WITH FOOD ALLERGIES

Vacations other than visiting family were a problem as I needed to cook almost every meal to be sure Rachel was safe. Fortunately, when our second daughter was born, Ed's distant cousin recommended a special vacation spot in Vermont called Smuggler's Notch Resort. This ski resort turned summer vacation wonderland rented us a three bedroom condo for the week. We shared it with Ed's parents. The condo had a fully stocked kitchen, including pots, pans, plates and utensils. Perfect. We just had to bring the food.

We started calling Smuggler's Notch "Smuggs" for short. The resort would turn into our second family home, and we became so spoiled that we refused to go on vacation anywhere else without having the facilities of a full kitchen or apartment. We packed a dry goods box for the road trip to Smuggs with all of the allergy safe substitute ingredients: Fleischmann's margarine (pareve), and Ener-G egg replacer; safe foods that were dairy and egg free like Teddy Grahams and rice cakes, made in a dairy free facility; soy yogurt in a cooler with ice; Rachel's fishy mask (Pulmicort). We needed to be organized and prepared for emergencies because Smuggs was a fairly remote location in Vermont. The nearest hospital was 45 minutes away by car.

Most families go out to dinner while on vacation. Not our family! Normally Rachel was able to eat a plain hamburger without the bun at a restaurant or a plain steak. But once, when we went to the resort restaurant that received most of its products from Cisco, she ordered a kids burger and vomited after we got back to the condo. This happened more than once.

Why?

We learned that burger and the kids' burger especially contained additives, one of which might have been "spices;" "spices" may have included mustard, which we later learned Rachel was allergic to. Unfortunately, the meat industry was not required to list specific spices on its packaging. For this reason, we could never be too careful. We learned to ask for 100% pure beef burgers.

PRESCHOOL
Rachel first started attending daycare when she was about 18 months old. She would go to the Mulberry Learning Center two days a week, and we would send her with a packed allergy-free lunch.

Rachel's second preschool was where I would eventually meet Melissa and Nancy, two friends who would lead me to connect with Rachel's Health Coach.

Having a food allergic child attend school was an effort for all involved. To keep Rachel safe, the subject of food allergies was an ongoing topic with the preschool teach-ers and other parents. It truly took a village to raise our food allergic child.

During school, the book series *Alexander the Elephant* empowered our daughter to explain her food allergies to her friends. She was extremely articulate for a pre-school kid and absolutely comfortable explaining what she could and could not eat. Her friends would ask at the lunch/snack table "Are you allergic to this or that? Are you allergic to water?" Rachel would confidently say "Yes" or "No."

One week when Rachel was in preschool, she was dubbed as the "Shabbat helper." When the kids in her school celebrated Shabbat, they lit candles, drank pre-tend wine or grape juice and ate a piece of braided bread called challah. Each child took turns being the Shabbat Helper in each classroom every Friday. This made Ra-chel feel special because she was able to pretend light the candles for her class at the end of the week, and I was invited in as a guest to help her. Then she was giv-en a cute little bag to bring home so she could pretend celebrate with toy candles, a wooden wine cup and a wooden challah.

This encouraged us to celebrate Shabbat at home. It was cute, but it wasn't necessarily part of our weekly ritual, as we weren't religious. The circumstance en-couraged me to learn how to make my own challah, a bread traditionally eaten on a Jewish holiday including Shabbat.

Rivka, another mom from Rachel's preschool, gave me her aunt's delicious egg free "water challah" recipe. I tried it from scratch. It came out OK for my first time, but then Ed suggested that I purchase a bread maker to make the dough, which I did. My husband the domestic became my ingenious savior. I learned how to substitute Ener-G egg replacer for the eggs and to add honey to the outside instead of using egg wash. Other ingredients in the challah were water, flour, yeast, salt, and sugar.

I could have spared myself all this work as there was one dairy free, nut free bakery that sold "water challah," but this bakery was out of the way. Besides, once I learned how to make my own with honey on top, my family loved *my* freshly baked challah! Plus, I could make a batch with four cups of flour, divide the dough, bake three loaves and freeze the other two for future weeks. Since we occasionally skipped a week, this allowed the three-hour baking operation to be conducted only once a month.

CHAPTER 7

New Avenues Opening Up

JANUARY 11, 2006

I was always searching for new ideas and possible answers to my food allergy questions. There had to be a better way! My friend Nancy was also looking for allergy solutions because her son had some serious digestive constraints. I remember she would go to Whole Foods and purchase special flour to make homemade muffins for her son with specific unprocessed ingredients. She became an allergy diet mentor to me and inspired me to try new recipes. Later, she would also be instrumental in finding the health practitioner that healed Rachel of her allergies.

EXPLORING ALTERNATIVE HEALING

In preschool, my daughter became friendly with Randi, another girl. Soon we became good friends with Randi's family, especially her mother Dee. We would often bring our daughters to the playground so they could play together.

Randi's family was very understanding of our food allergy issues; Dee was allergic to mushrooms and tomatoes. During playdates, Dee and I would talk about many things. Among them was what was safe for Rachel to eat, Dee's symptoms from her allergies, such as migraines, and how she finally figured out what was causing them.

And this is where our story changes. Dee told me she had worked with someone to help release her from her food allergies. One part of her therapy was to hold the allergy-causing ingredients in her hand; this was meant to desensitize her system and eliminate the allergy. She didn't find it effective, but nevertheless this is how I was introduced to NAET, a form of energy medicine.

Discovered by Dr. Devi S. Nambudripad in 1983, NAET is a non-invasive, drug free, natural solution to alleviate allergies of all types and intensities. It implements a blend of selective energy balancing, testing and treatment procedures from acupuncture/acupressure, allopathy, chiropractic, nutritional, and kinesiological disciplines of medicine.

NAET has been shown to successfully alleviate adverse reactions in some people to egg, milk, peanuts, penicillin, aspirin, mushrooms, shellfish, latex, grass, ragweed, flowers, perfume, animal dander, animal epithelial, make-up, chemicals, cigarette smoke, pathogens, heat, cold, and other environmental agents.

One allergen is treated at a time. Some with mild immune compromise may need just one treatment to desensitize one allergen. Others with more severe immune deficiencies may take 15-20 office visits to desensitize a severe allergen.

While NAET doesn't work for everyone, including Dee, energy medicine would work for Rachel!

CHAPTER 8

More Troubling Incidents

NEW DAY CAMP: SUMMER 2008

Once Rachel graduated from preschool, we sent her to a new summer day camp. The camp employed a wonderful director who completely understood food allergies as she had a son with anaphylactic peanut allergies who at the time was 24 years old, alive and well.

One day Rachel attended a cooking class at camp. I remember the date distinctly: Monday July 7th, 2008. I completely trusted the Director because of her years of experience as a director and as a mother with a child of food allergies. She knew what she was doing. Rachel needed to avoid eggs, dairy, and nuts, and another kid in the group was allergic to wheat.

The camp Director purposely bought pancake mix from Whole Foods with kamut flour to be sure both of the allergic children in the group were safe. I was in the exercise room, in the same building as the camp when my cell phone rang. "Hello, Mrs. Bassin, Rachel has hives on her upper legs..."

"I'll be right there!" I exclaimed as I jumped off the elliptical machine.

The camp nurse was not in that day, but I trusted the Director. Honestly, she knew what she was doing. We went into the nurse's office to retrieve Rachel's personal stash of Benadryl from the medical cabinet, and after giving Rachel the appropriate dosage we called the doctor's office to receive further instructions.

We were problem solving. What could have happened? I went into the kitchen and read all of the ingredients on the labels, but could not figure out what might have caused an allergic reaction. The doctor told us to take her to the hospital for observation.

The director suggested I take her myself. Since she was fine, she didn't need an ambulance to take her to the hospital. On the way, I kept an EpiPen in hand and kept a conversation going to make sure her breathing was normal, while continuing glancing at her to see if she had any more hives. The hospital observed her for several hours and put her on Prednisolone for two days. We then made an appointment with Rachel's new allergist.

I went to Whole Foods to get another package of the same pancake mix that the camp director used in the cooking class to see if perhaps it was a fluke. I tried making the same pancake product at home to see if there was some type of cross contact issue in the camp kitchen. I gave Rachel a plate of the pancakes made in my allergy free kitchen with the new bag of pancake mix. Rachel smelled these pancakes and said she was allergic to them. She was that sensitive and we trusted her instincts.

The allergist did more skin tests which were positive for mustard, and pancake mix which contained kamut, oat, and soy. Apparently the kamut, an Egyptian organic grain, was the problem. The allergist determined that we should now be avoiding kamut. That seemed easy enough.

TRYING PROBIOTICS

Five days after this incident, Rachel's stomach hurt all night and she was twitching in bed. We gave her acidophilus – a probiotic – and lots of water. I was taking probiotics reactively instead of proactively, so we had them in the house.

This was the first time we ever gave them to Rachel. They were pills, so it was hard to get her to swallow them, but they were very small and now she was old enough to learn. We never thought to look for a child/kid version of probiotics, and none of the physicians we ever worked with ever suggested it. But I was running out of ideas and things to try. If her stomach hurt, perhaps she was constipated and it might help.

Regretfully, this was a one-time incident. We did not continue to give probiotics to Rachel. Little did I know at this point that probiotics, by providing the gut with healthy bacteria is not only the secret to a healthy gut and therefore a healthy immune system, but that it was the destruction of Rachel's good gut flora from long-term antibiotics that had much to do with her poor immune system and food allergies.

JOYS AND PERILS OF SCHOOL:
SEPTEMBER 2008

Rachel was now five. She loved dressing up as a princess and was learning how to ride a two-wheeler bike. Smart and quick, she was ahead of others her age in learning how to read. She loved listening to stories. Every night we would lie in bed and read to her for 45 minutes at a time, and if we stopped to take just one breath or moisten our palate, she would jab us in the arm and say "Just READ!" In spite of food allergies, illness, scary trips to the emergency room and being restricted from eating what others were eating, she had confidence and a strong sense of self.

At the end of preschool in an interview, Rachel said:

"I like to ride my bike, pick flowers, go to the beach and build sand castles. My favorite color is orange, purple, pink. My favorite food is spaghetti. I love eating soy ice cream sandwiches. When I grow up I want to be a princess or a queen."

That's my girl!

Our little princess was excited about going to kindergarten. She looked forward to waiting at the bus stop each morning with the rest of her neighborhood friends.

Nevertheless, kindergarten was an adjustment for me even more than for Rachel. The warm and fuzzy preschool environment where I could walk into the building, talk to the teachers face to face and hug them was over. Now the bus would pick her up, drop her off and bring her home while she spent the day with educators who didn't have the same caring and loving investment in her as had her preschool teachers.

ALLERGY BRACELET
Ed and I had to figure out how to keep Rachel out of harm's way as we could no longer control her environment.

Upon recommendation from the pediatrician, I purchased two pink Vital ID bracelets. They were especially helpful once Rachel started going on drop-off playdates. Since we would not always be with her, it was important that her medical information and our contact information was always on her wrist.

EDUCATING THE SCHOOL STAFF
The next thing I had to do was to ensure that the school environment was safe.

I needed to be sure the teachers were trained on allergy awareness and EpiPen procedures. I needed to know that the nurse had my contact information in an emergency and the necessary medications on hand. I had to find out where Rachel would eat and how the cafeteria would be managed during lunch to keep her safe. All this proved to be a challenge. Though I'm certain that Rachel was not the first child to have food allergies, the school seemed uninformed and not helpful in providing information about how we would keep her safe.

My cool-as-a-cucumber husband didn't have my worries. He believed that the school system could handle it and discouraged me from making too much of a stink. Pick my battles carefully, he advised. Luckily I kept this in mind when I went to the open house before school started; when I tried to talk with Rachel's new teacher Mrs. Taylor about how she managed food allergies in the classroom, she ignored me! She thought I was a crazy parent. I was horrified at her lack of concern. This was going to be an uphill battle.

Fortunately, I could control the food Rachel ate for lunch. Kindergarten in our town was only a half day because of space and funding limitations. Rachel went to morning kindergarten. In the afternoon, we enrolled her in an after school education program three days a week. This program happened to be in the elementary school building, so Rachel would bring her lunch to school Monday, Tuesday, and Thursday. On Wednesday, she would take the "mint day" as she would call it, or the 'midday' bus home. On Wednesday, we would have lunch together.

I filled out all of the appropriate school forms that the school nurse required, informed her of Rachel's allergies, and brought in Benadryl and an EpiPen to keep in her office. As it had only been a couple of months since Rachel had an allergic reaction to an unknown allergen (kamut flour), and we had no idea what else she might be allergic to that might come up in a new environmental setting, we wanted her fully prepared.

I called the bus company to find out how they would handle an anaphylactic reaction on the bus. The director told me no food was allowed to be eaten on the bus.

In addition to keeping Rachel safe at school, I also had to keep her safe on Friday, as she was signed up for a Shabbat Club program with her pre-school friends. The other parents and I would carpool to this program. She needed to bring her lunch with her, even though all the other kids would have pizza. It was okay as we were used to Rachel bringing her own food everywhere she went and she didn't seem to mind. After all, she knew what her body felt like when she had an allergic reaction and that we were taking the proper precautions to avoid these scary incidents.

What a trooper! I was so proud of her resilience and great attitude.

SOME LINGERING CONCERNS
Rachel was doing well in Mrs. Taylor's class. She LOVED school! Nevertheless, I still had some concerns.

Two weeks after school started, I sent an e-mail to the nurse.

Issue #1: Scrounge project. The kids took garbage or items that you would normally put in your recycling bin at home like milk carton jugs, mayonnaise jars, yogurt containers, etc... and brought them into school to build abstract art in the classroom. Rachel was allergic to many of these recyclable items! Even if well cleaned them, the tiniest molecule could potentially cause a life-threatening allergic reaction. I wanted to know how the teacher would prevent such an incident, and I needed the nurse to address the possible ramifications of the "scrounge" project.

As Rachel wanted to participate, the nurse and I decided it would be okay if all "scrounge" items were either non-food items like newspaper, paper towel rolls, or simple packaging materials, or if the items were placed in the dishwasher before they entered the classroom. This worked fine and Rachel participated without an issue.

Issue#2: Hand washing: Hand sanitizer was used in the classroom as the primary source of cleanliness before and after snacks. And though I lauded the school for doing this, it was still a problem for Rachel. While hand sanitizer would kill germs, food allergies are proteins and good old soap and water was a much better way to clean hands in the classroom. The custodian fixed the faucet in the classroom so that it worked properly and Mrs. Taylor and her class were able to use the sink to wash their hands before and after snacks.

Issue#3: Eating snack on the rug in the class-room. The teacher insisted that the kids eat snack on the rug in the classroom. I was appalled! The rug could not be cleaned. What if someone spilled milk or yogurt on the rug? That allergen would be in the carpet the entire year. The nurse suggested that Rachel bring in a plastic sit-up-on like they did in girl scouts when she was a girl. I didn't think this was a good idea because it would single Rachel out among her friends and I didn't want her to be isolated.

I tried to get the teacher to feed the kids at the tables, but Mrs. Taylor needed this time to prepare for her next lesson and use of the tables was part of the lesson plan. We tried designating one table for Rachel and her friends, but this solution was short lived because the kids wanted to all eat together. I cautioned Rachel not to touch any-thing she was allergic to and to be careful.

Fortunately, we survived the year without any major allergic reactions, but I was on pins and needles the entire year.

FIRST GRADE: SEPTEMBER 2009
By the time Rachel started first grade, we had moved across town. Rachel went to another grammar school in the new school district. This school's nurse and teacher were much more cooperative. Plus we had one year of kindergarten under our belts without any reac-

tions. We started to feel a little more confident with the school system, especially with Rachel's personal supply of antihistamine and epinephrine in the nurse's office. Fortunately, she did not need to use them.

OVERNIGHT CAMP WEEKEND TRY-OUT: SUMMER 2010

Our next challenge came the following summer when Rachel went to overnight camp. I was opposed to the idea initially because I thought it would be too risky considering her food allergies. But my husband, who never went to overnight camp, thought it would be a great experience for our girls. Rachel, now 7 years old, wanted to go, even without knowing any of the other kids in the "try it out" program.

After I spoke with the camp director and thoroughly informed her of how to manage Rachel's allergies, Ed and I gave our okay as it was only for two nights. When we told Rachel the good news, she was overcome with joy at the opportunity of making more friends and practicing her ever-growing independence. Still, she was naïve and didn't know how to take care of herself in an emergency situation. We would rely on the camp to make good judgements in the dining hall and during any unforeseen signs of an allergic reaction.

That proved to be a mistake.

With some trepidation, on Friday night we dropped her off at the designated parking lot. She settled in quickly and chatted away. The kids watched the Disney movie *Hercules* on the bus, and Rachel loved it.

That night we received an email from the Camp Director: "Hi Holli and Ed, We have had a great first day at camp! While you were wondering what we were doing, we were getting to know each other and camp-what a great tour, going for a motorboat ride, going for a swim, celebrating Shabbat, eating chicken patty sandwiches, turkey and challah...oh and lots of vegetables! Tonight we are going to sing our hearts out and then go to bed by 9 p.m. It has been a great and busy day and we are all looking forward to another day at camp tomorrow. Stay warm tonight."

When we viewed the pictures on line, Rachel looked tired but all was okay. One huge sigh of relief!

On Sunday afternoon we picked her up at the camp. The director approached us and told us that Rachel threw up the day before. Even worse, one of the counselors took me aside and reported "the third time she threw up, she made it to the garbage can."

Apparently, someone inadvertently gave her a plate of egg pasta that she willingly ate. Initially, the camp did not recognize the vomiting as an allergic reaction, so no one bothered to call me to let me know she was sick. They hydrated her in the infirmary and sent her back to camp.

In the car on the way home, Rachel slept and in the same day developed a 102° fever. The triage nurse in our pediatric office assured us that the fever was unrelated to the vomiting and allergic reaction. I had my doubts. The body only has one immune system and the fever indicated it was clearly compromised.

Rachel said that the egg pasta tasted good, but that it wasn't worth getting sick!

I was furious: at the camp, and at myself for allowing this to happen. We wrote a lengthy letter to the head honcho of the camping organization. Within a day or two he called me. "A serious issue is a serious issue!" he said with apology. Nevertheless, we never sent her to that camp again.

THE PEANUT CHALLENGE

When Rachel was seven years old, the results of her skin tests for peanut and tree nut were low enough for a food challenge. We were always vigilant about avoiding these allergens, so as far as we know, she never had any accidental exposure, but we needed to check to be sure.

I was told to bring in peanut butter, but the allergist was not satisfied with the brand that we purchased. She said it was produced in a facility with other tree nuts, so she condescendingly stated that we could use the brand from the hospital cafeteria or not do the test.

The peanut butter was carefully measured; we spent four hours in the hospital doctor's office while she ate small increasing amounts of the peanut butter in half hour increments. In the end we had good news: we were given the go-ahead to start eating peanuts. We were to incorporate them into Rachel's diet and be sure that she ate them a few times a week as not to lose her peanut tolerance. I soon found a new snack that she could eat – Bomba! I found it in the kosher section of a supermarket in Brookline. This was the snack that would instigate the entire *Learning Early About Peanut Allergy* or LEAP Study which would be published in a few years. The study would be a randomized controlled clinical trial designed and conducted by the Immune Tolerant Network (ITN) to determine the best strategy to prevent peanut allergy in young children.

My daughter loved Bomba! It was a puffy snack with peanut on the outside. We bought it by the caseload on Amazon. Unfortunately she was not able to bring it to camp that year because so many other kids had peanut allergies. This didn't seem to bother Rachel because she would be just so excited to go to camp.

About a month after the peanut challenge, we went back for an almond challenge.

I purchased the appropriate almond butter recommended by the allergist and we spent another 4 hours in the clinical setting of the doctor's office. This location was in case Rachel needed immediate medical attention. If need be, we could easily be moved to the emergency room. During the food challenge, Rachel ate small, increasing amounts of almond butter every half hour or so. At the end of the four hour period, we were sent home. We passed!!!

This was life changing!!!

After Rachel outgrew her nut allergy, we started drinking almond milk instead of soy milk. I really liked it! I thought it tasted much better than cow's milk, which we still were terrified to have in the house, or soy milk, which we were ready for a change from.

We also started incorporating new things into her diet, like Luna bars.

PASSOVER: APRIL 2011

When Ed's nephew, Ben was eight years old, he flew by himself to visit his Uncle Ed in Boston. Now that Rachel was eight years old, it was family tradition for a niece or nephew to visit their aunt and uncle. We agreed to send Rachel to Pittsburgh during the week of Passover, which also happened to be a school vacation week. Rachel was excited to see her grandparents, cousins, aunt and uncle, and she greatly looked forward to the trip. Once again she had the opportunity to separate from her parents. Looking forward to expressing her sense of freedom and independence with her extended family, she bravely flew by herself as an unaccompanied minor. When she stepped off the plane, her doting grandparents and loving aunt greeted her with open arms.

Even though she was with family, who of course would do everything to keep her safe, I was beside myself with apprehension. This trip was during Passover, the "egg eating" Jewish holiday -- and Rachel was allergic to eggs and dairy! At home, I was vigilant and my kitchen was allergy safe; we never let anything she would eat touch these allergens. I sent her with the faith that this could be done at my sister-in-law's house as well. Also, she would staying with "Aunt Minty" -- named as such by Rachel because she grew so many mints in her garden. Aunt Minty kept a kosher kitchen, so she was very much aware of any foods that contained dairy ingredients and she was also a medical doctor.

To prepare my sister-in-law for Rachel's arrival, Ed spoke with his sister to ensure proper care would be taken regarding food. She agreed to set aside a convenient safe place in the kitchen to keep foods Rachel could eat without any cross contact.

A week prior to Rachel's trip, we shipped a box with some packaged foods of things she was used to eating. I emailed Aunt Minty a detailed list of Rachel's menu (see Appen-dix B). And, importantly, we sent along liquid Benadryl, EpiPen and Rachel's inhalers...for emergency use.

Gratefully, there was only one small incident when Aunt Minty needed to administer a small dose of antihistamine for a minor reaction. But overall all went smoothly and Rachel had a great time. She especially enjoyed going to the Science Museum.

For me, though it was an ordeal. Besides the prior year's disastrous overnight weekend at camp, this was the second time Rachel was away from us and she was gone for an entire week!

And there was very little communication with my sister-in-law who was too busy for chatty conversations and not a phone person. I did speak with Rachel on the phone to verify she was doing well, but I wanted more details than an eight-year old could provide. The adult level of communication was missing.

I also missed Rachel terribly, and felt as if someone had cut off my left arm. But this visit prepared me for the lack of communication I would have with her when she went to overnight camp in a few years.

EPINEPHRINE INCIDENT#2:
ACCIDENTAL EXPOSURE IN SCHOOL

Rachel had now gone to overnight camp, spent a week with our family in Pittsburgh and had survived most of the year in school without any anaphylactic re-actions. Thank goodness! I was beginning to feel more confident that we could prevent accidental exposures when Rachel was away from us to keep her safe. That was until June 15, 2011, the last day of school.

The day before school ended, I went into the nurse's office to pick up Rachel's EpiPen and other incidentals. She didn't need it all year, and the next day was only a half day.

The last day of school was miserably hot and the kids were thirsty. A well-meaning volunteer brought some popsicles into my daughter's second grade classroom.

I had finished my morning and was just getting out of the shower when the phone rang. "Hello, Mrs. Bassin."

"Yes,"

"This is Alison from Rachel's school. The nurse just administered an EpiPen to your daughter and the ambulance is on its way. Do you want to meet them at the hospital or come to the school?"

"No. I'll be right there."

I quickly dressed, ran out the door and arrived at the school before the ambulance pulled away. I was in a panicked state, but remained calm and in control. I needed to investigate the situation. Rachel was only at the beginning of anaphylactic shock. She vomited in the nurse's office, had that sense of panic or "doom" as it's described and broke out with a few hives. Fortunately, her breathing was not yet compromised. I hopped onto the ambulance that was still in the school parking lot and spoke with the paramedic while Rachel was lying there on the stretcher.

The nurse had given Rachel an EpiPen and the Paramedic was adamant about the fact that he did not believe Rachel was in anaphylactic shock. He said anaphylaxis is breathing related and she was not having trouble breathing. Then he said she just got nervous because she ate something that she was allergic to. He basically undermined Rachel's opinion of what was happening to her own body! I explained that vomiting is just one symptom of an allergic reaction that can easily and quickly be escalated to an anaphylactic reaction.

I assured the paramedic that this was a serious incident and that the nurse had indeed followed protocol by giving her an EpiPen. I was appalled at the paramedic's unprofessionalism and couldn't believe I was having this conversation with him in the ambulance while my daughter was lying there on a stretcher!

With the kindergarten teacher at my side comforting me, I stood shaking as I watched Rachel being driven away in the ambulance.

OMG!

As I knew she was now under medical supervision, I didn't go with her because I wanted to read the ingredient list on the popsicle box before going to the hospital. As you may recall, Rachel had another allergic reaction to popsicles when she was two. I also wanted to keep the box in case I would ever need it for any reason and to read the label.

I ended up spending four hours in the emergency room as the medical team observed Rachel to be certain that she did not have any more reactions once the EpiPen and Benadryl wore off. Luckily she was fine.

But it was very scary and I felt traumatized for days. My amazing trooper quickly recovered, and when we got home she ate a normal dinner.

Once we were home, the teacher and the volunteer came to our house with flowers to visit Rachel and make sure she was OK. I told them how the food sensitivities started in infancy and how thankful I was that she was still alive and graduating from second grade. I also received several e-mails from concerned parents for which I was grateful.

SCHOOL RESPONSE
As it turned out, the popsicles that were brought in on the last day of school contained milk and no one checked to see if Rachel was allergic. I did not even know that they were going to be serving popsicles on the last day of school. Anyway, Rachel trusted the adults in the room and ate 1/4 of one.

When we leave children at school under their supervision, we hold the school responsible for keeping our children safe. Food allergies in children is not a rare event. Approximately one in every thirteen children under 18 years of age in the U.S. have food allergies. That's roughly two in every classroom whose life may be threatened by the ingestion or exposure to dairy, eggs, fish, shellfish, peanuts, tree nuts, soy, wheat, and other foods. Schools need to be fully prepared for the possibility of a life threatening incident and take maximum precautions.

Rachel's teacher *was* fully aware of the situation and the need for extreme caution as to what Rachel ate or was exposed to. But on a momentous occasion such as the last day of school, something slipped through the cracks and he failed in his responsibilities. I was irate and felt all involved should take responsibility. Ed had advised me to pick my battles and here was my chance. And so, while I was grateful for the amount of concern I received from the school and parents, I wrote the following letter to the Principal of the school to insure that this would never happen again. After thanking them for their quick response, I wrote:

"Communication was definitely lacking prior to the incident. A second adult never verified that the popsicles were safe for Rachel to eat, and I did not know they were being supplied. What is the exact protocol for food in the classroom at our school? I do not believe there was any notice, e-mail or communication sent home prior to the accidental exposure on the last day of school.

During a situation such as this, there are many variables beyond our control, one of which is the labeling of allergy information on food products. In this incident, the label on the box did not have the modern "food allergy label" with the most common allergen ingredients such as milk bolded and/or the words: "Allergens" or "Allergy Statement" on the packaging.

However, the words "milkfat" and "nonfat milk" were clearly on the ingredients list along with "whey" and "whey protein" which are also dairy protein ingredients, and to which Rachel is therefore allergic."

The Principal called me the next day. He applauded my attitude in turning this into a learning experience and assured me that safety measures would be heightened in the school. After that day, I noticed extreme vigilance when food was brought into the school for either of my daughters.

I've since received many emails or notes requiring my response. For example, if the school is going to provide chocolate chip cookies in the classroom, the teacher will send me an e-mail with the ingredient list. Or if they expect to have food in the science room, a letter will go home that I need to sign before my daughter can participate in the project. Or on a field day, a note will go out to all parents with labels and ingredients of all food that will be available and I usually need to sign it.

I contacted the popsicle manufacturer, who denied any fault or blame. The woman stated that the popsicle box was appropriately labeled with the milk ingredient according to FDA labeling laws. The company then sent me several free coupons for ice cream snacks that I donated to the local food pantry.

I also visited with the Fire Department to explain anaphylaxis vs. allergic reaction. In response, I received a call from the Medical Director of the Fire Department. I repeated with him the conversation I had with the paramedic in the ambulance. He thanked me for my comments and concerns and assured me that the town would address the issue. I didn't follow up again after his call.

A VISIT WITH GRANDMA: JULY 2011

After two incidents where the EpiPen had to be used, one at home and one at school, I felt more anxious than ever about staying close to Rachel at all times in the event of another anaphylactic incident. But life must go on and Ed and I planned a trip to Reno – just the two of us without the girls. My mother, who lives in New Jersey, graciously volunteered to care for her granddaughters while we were away. I trusted my mother because she had cared for Rachel and Iris many times before and she was well aware of how to manage Rachel's food allergies.

All of us were excited about the trip. My mother would get to see her granddaughters, the girls would spend some quality time with their grandmother, and Ed and I would get some time together by ourselves – something all couples need.

And so we drove the girls to NJ and then took a flight to Reno.

Here are the safe foods that my mother had available for Rachel.

ALMOND MILK
Rachel liked Blue Diamond Almond Breeze milk.

PEANUT BUTTER AND JELLY
Rachel was eating the "Skippy natural with honey" peanut butter and grape, strawberry, or blueberry jelly. I did not specify the brand of jelly my mother needed to buy because we never had a cross contact issue with any of these products. My mother knew what kind of bread to buy, and I would check the labels before we left.

REPLACEMENT BUTTER
Since dairy was not allowed in Rachel's diet, my mother needed to buy instead Fleischmann's unsalted Ⓤpareve margarine sticks. These margarine sticks were labeled in green, while the original dairy version had a red label.

MEAT
My mother wanted to buy turkey breast or deli meat, but a lot of the deli meat had spices. As "spices" could be another word for mustard, we didn't want to take the chance. Plus deli meat contained other bad stuff like chemicals and we tried to stay away from the processed meats. I advised my mother to go to the deli counter and have them slice the less-processed thanksgiving turkey breast or roast beef that they made in the store.

BAGEL
Rachel could have any bagel except egg. Blueberry and cinnamon raisin were her favorite flavors, either

with jelly or plain. The same was true for Iris, except Iris would eat cream cheese.

PASTA
Rachel could eat pasta without eggs, and I suggested that my mother put some olive oil on it or just leave it plain. I told her if she bought a box of pasta, I would check the label.

CHICKEN NUGGETS
Rachel enjoyed chicken nuggets, and we bought the Empire brand.

OTHER THINGS ON THE LIST
In addition, we brought to NJ: Luna Bars for breakfast; Fiber One hamburger buns; some additional snacks for the girls; and two EpiPens and Benadryl just in case!

While we were in Reno, I called to check in with my mother every day. I got details on what the kids did, ate, and how well they slept; probably too much detail in Ed's opinion, but it was all good. Everyone was happy!

Fortunately, no incidents occurred at Grandma Camp, a huge success for all. Plus Ed and I had a great time in Reno.

NEW CAMPER WEEKEND:
OCTOBER 2011 (3ᴿᴰ GRADE)
Despite our bad experience at the try-it-out camper weekend the previous summer and the allergic reaction

on the last day of school, Rachel wanted to go to overnight camp. What an adventurer was our daughter. She strove for that sense of independence.

And so, in the summer of 2011, we went "camp shopping" and decided to give it another try. This time we did our homework and visited about five additional overnight camps. Some camps tried to sell themselves to potential campers by being nut-free, but nut-free didn't help us because Rachel had outgrown her nut allergy and actually needed to eat nuts in order to stay tolerant to them.

We finally made a decision and, as the new camp had a new camper weekend in the fall, we signed Rachel up for the weekend. Initially we were concerned that she would attend without knowing anyone, but as it turned out, a friend's two daughters who we knew from our vacations in Vermont would also be joining her.

One of the sisters arrived at the weekend cabin before we did, and since the younger sister and our daughter were assigned to the same cabin, her friend was able to save Rachel a bed. They would be sleeping next to each other. It was heartwarming that there was someone Rachel knew – even another 8 year old – to look out for her.

We ate dinner with the kids Friday night before leaving Rachel for the weekend – one less meal she had to eat without my supervision. I was able to observe the dining hall procedure. The director took Rachel into the kitchen and had her speak directly with the chef. This chef was our savoir! At every meal, she and the chef determined what food was safe for her to eat. Other kids went into the kitchen on the other side to get a cart of food for their table. This would be OK. Rachel would have direct communication with the chef, and she would be able to develop a relationship with him.

With our fingers crossed, we drove home with our younger daughter.

The weekend turned out to be a success, but I still was unconvinced that this was the summer to begin sending Rachel to overnight camp.

NEW CAMPER WEEKEND: OCTOBER 2012
When Rachel was in 4th grade, we decided to try one more weekend at the camp she would eventually be attending. If this turned out to be a success and the camp was confident they could manage her food allergies during the busy summer season, we would consider signing her up for the following summer.

At this point our younger daughter was in second grade and would be eligible for the 10- day program that following summer. However, our Rachel was too old for the 10- day program, and we had no choice but to send her for the entire four-week session. Our younger daughter wanted to go on the weekend that October, but she was a little more anxious about it than her sister. Having her big sister on campus would be comforting even if she would not be in the same cabin.

We drove both daughters the two-hour distance to the camp, dropped them off for the weekend, and returned on Sunday to pick them up.

The weekend was a success! Rachel met two girls who would become two lifelong friends, Jolie and Emily, both from New York.

Most importantly, no food allergy incidents! It was time to sign the girls up for overnight camp the next summer.

HARRY POTTER SLEEPUNDER: MAY 12, 2012

When my food-allergic daughter turned nine, we had a very elaborate Harry Potter sleep-under. A sleep under is a birthday party where the kids play games, watch a movie, have cake, possibly put on their PJ's and then go home. It's like a sleepover without the sleep or breakfast part. There were tons of ideas on the Internet and award-winning parties to emulate. I sent out invitations by owl mail:

Dear Miss _____,

"We are pleased to inform you that you have been accepted at Hogwart's School of Witchcraft and Wizardry. A special pre-term belated birthday sleep under celebration will be held on Saturday, May 12th at 5:00p.m. In honor of our newest Head Girl, Miss Bassin.

Please RSVP by owl e-mail (insert my email address), or by Muggle phone at (insert phone number) by Sunday May 6th.

Transportation to Hogwarts will depart from King's Cross Station, Our address, Gate 9 3/4. Activities will include games and the viewing of Harry Potter and the Prisoner of Azkaban.

The menu will include Magic Potions, Heavy Appetizers, Forbidden Forest Fruit, Popcorn, Cauldron Cake, Bertie Bott's Every Flavor Beans and Drooble's Best Blowing Gum.

Wizard or Muggle (non-wizard) attire are appropriate.

Term will end at approximately 8:30 p.m.

Yours Sincerely,

Edward and Holli Bassin
Deputy Headmaster and Headmistress"

We bought a sorting hat and put a cell phone under it, our clever way to sort the girls into different houses. My husband went into the attic and called from another phone, and his voice spoke through the hat! The kids were mesmerized.

We set up a Quidditch field in our backyard equipped with a snitch, and the kids brought broomsticks. Once again, I used the castle cake pan. This time I mixed the appropriate colors and used them to transform the cake into a Hogwarts castle.

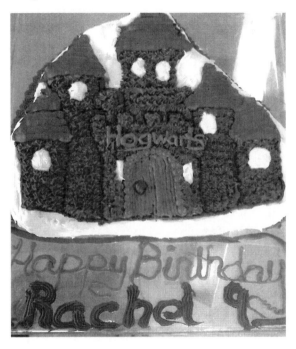

The Wilton castle cake pan transformed from Disney to The Prisoner of Azkaban. I made allergy-free bread dough in the bread maker and rolled the dough into breadsticks that we called wands. I made chicken drumsticks in the oven and turned them into magic dragon legs, and we bought non-allergic jelly beans for a Bertie Bott's touch.

The party was a magical success.

NEW CAKE-MAKING SAVIOR

The Hogwarts Castle was probably the last elaborate cake that I made. Business owners were starting to see the need for allergy-free products, and lucky for me the time had come that a local bakery started baking allergy-free cupcakes. Though expensive, they saved me hours of work. The bakery's cupcake business soon expanded to a cake business. I had a new cake making savior!

They were located just a few stores away from an ice cream parlor, so we would sometimes walk into town for a cupcake outing with friends, giving them a choice of treats. Down the road, we would be able to go into this cupcake store and order cupcakes with real buttercream, but this wasn't even in the realm of possibilities... at least not yet!

Addressing food allergy issues from an etiquette standpoint was becoming easier because I was more comfortable speaking with friends and family about these issues. I learned that the main focus of a social gathering was not about the food. It was about the company we were with, and overall enjoyment of the celebration.

To provide positive examples for my daughter and be a role model for her, I started volunteering to bring dessert to other kids' parties so that I knew my daughter could eat the cake. I made a cake for our summer block party and another for an informal group boating outing/picnic. This way most everyone could eat the cake and we could all feel like we were enjoying the celebration together without having to be interrupted by what knife touched what piece of cake.

PART TWO
TRANSITION PERIOD

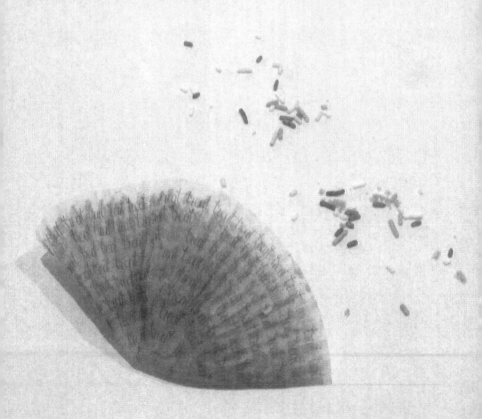

CHAPTER 9

Professional Career

Prior to Rachel's birth, I worked as a Human Resources Manager for Atabok, a small digital asset management company in Newton, MA. This start-up company managed secure data solutions for internet communications. Their software encrypted data, and their e-mail system was very cool. You could send an e-mail and then decide to retrieve it back and delete it, or you could have the data deleted after a specified period of time.

As the sole member of the HR department, I worked with upper management to help build the company in two locations, both in Newton, MA. One location housed the software engineering department, and the other was for corporate operations. I created and implemented compensation programs, developed processes, and in just a few months grew the employee population from 42 to 56.

After September 11, 2001, the business changed. We lost funding, and our sales department was underperforming their revenue goals. The company had to downsize; I was directly involved with managing the employee exit process. We brought the payroll down to 25 employees, and it was no secret that my job was on the line. For the last trimester of my pregnancy I was underemployed, and subsequently laid off after my maternity leave. My husband and I joked that I would be going on *eternity leave*.

As a newborn infant, Rachel was my new boss, keeping me busy and sleep deprived. But I needed intellectual stimulation and, for the first time experienced the motherly dilemma of wanting to be at work, yet wanting to be with my baby. The solution? A job that provided a work-life balance – easier said than done.

And then the opportunity arose. Ed, who had a PhD in sociology and prior experience with Episode Treatment Groups (ETG's) and Stata Programming, was growing his own software company. ProfSoft paid royalties to another software company called Symmetry Health Data Systems, Inc. This software was embedded into the ProfSoft software that grouped data, and the ProfSoft software analyzed the data. Ed needed help with the bookkeeping, hiring and other organizational projects. I said "Why not let me do it?" and of course he hired me.

While Rachel was a baby, I worked at ProfSoft on a part- time basis. It was a perfect arrangement. The company office was located in the walk-out basement of our house, and I could work while Rachel was napping. One of the guys I worked with at Atabok referred to Ed as "The Man in the Basement." We also had a separate entrance for Bongani, the new software programmer that I recruited and hired.

Business was going well for Profsoft and so was our arrangement. As we were working at home, Rachel could be with us when necessary when we were both working. Bongani adored our cute little toddler. One day, to his amusement, Rachel climbed up on his lap and insisted that he find Elmo on his computer.

SELLING THE FAMILY BUSINESS

Soon after Iris was born, ProfSoft grew too big for the operation to run out of the basement of our home. We moved the office to a building on the other side of town; it was still close enough to work with two small children at home. We hired a nanny whom we shared with another family. Maria worked for us two days per week so I could go into the office. She was like a member of the family and stayed with us for five years until just before the first day of kindergarten and second grade respectively. Sadly, she died in 2010 from complications of non-Hodgkin's lymphoma, an awful loss for our family.

In the fall of 2009, the industry was changing and we sold our business. I was devastated. I had been working at ProfSoft for six years in what I felt was a perfect work/life balance. The new company that bought

ProfSoft would no longer need a part-time Human Resources Manager. I was out of a job and Ed's job was changing from business owner of a small company to employee of a large company. On top of it, we were selling our house, building a new house, and moving to the other side of town.

Each one of these things was stressful in and of itself. Altogether, our lives were a total stress case. My body reacted and I had an emergency appendectomy.

Things started to calm in 2010, after we moved and settled, but I was still feeling a powerful need to have a career. So I started a new consulting business that involved recruiting and HR Consulting work for a few small companies in the Transitional Health Care and Intangible Asset industries. I also volunteered at a Human Resources professional organization and worked on their spring conference.

But the timing was poor for me to have started my consulting business. The economy was in an economic downturn, plus the ebbs and flows did not coincide with our family lifestyle.

And so by 2012 I felt that I needed something different. I started working with a professional Career Coach who strongly encouraged me to look into other avenues. As much of my life revolved around food allergies, I volunteered at the local office of a national non-profit allergy organization. One day the training director handed me a book written by an allergic person. She asked me to read it and write a review for their next newsletter.

The book intrigued me. *Maybe I should become an allergy coach.* I had enough experience!

I contacted several people who were doing this work and conducted informational interviews. And then I formed my company with my brand name: *Your Food Allergy Coach.*

I had a lot of work to do! I used 99designs.com to find someone to design and implement my website. On Rachel's 10th birthday I launched yourfoodallergycoach.com. Rachel and I were more tied at the hip than ever!

I started working with clients and developed an online presence. Then one day, my marketing coach encouraged me to write a blog post and I blew him away! I started writing articles such as "Sending Your Food Allergic Child to Camp," and "Traveling to Your Vacation Destination." Rachel, who's reading level was off the charts, read everything I wrote.

TRAINING OTHERS

In September 2013 I started conducting staff training programs for preschool and religious schools on managing food allergies in the classroom and keeping food allergic kids safe. Encouraging the schools to allocate time for training was a great way to provide food allergy awareness.

I used some of the resources on AllergyHome.org and immersed myself in this material. I found the *Living Confidently Handbook* by Anaphylaxis Canada and other well- known allergists immensely helpful when working with parents and staff.

My training workshop included FDA food labeling laws, reading labels, avoiding cross-contact in the classroom, signs and symptoms of anaphylaxis, and how to activate an emergency action plan. As a non-medical professional, I was not qualified to conduct EpiPen training, so I showed a video published by the drug company and provided training tools for staff to practice. I received very positive feedback such as:

"Speaker was informative and knowledgeable. Training was interactive with great conversation."

"I applaud you and your family. It's amazing how you choose to take your time to educate and advocate for others."

"I found the training to be very helpful and informative. Looking at and comparing food labels was VERY eye opening."

"I liked hearing your personal accounts. As a parent who hasn't had to deal with this first hand, it really helps me empathize with those that do."

I was now a food allergy mom pro. Not only had we adjusted to Rachel's food allergies so that life seemed relatively normal, but I was now using my experience to teach others. I had found my niche.

CHAPTER 10

What's in a Label?

Now 9 years old, Rachel had not had an allergic episode since the last day of second grade. And so, while Ed and I were of course always vigilant about reading labels and avoiding eggs, dairy, kamut flour, garlic and mustard, her most prominent allergens, we now felt relaxed enough to enjoy life as a family. With this carefree attitude, all four of us decided to go for a bike ride on a beautiful warm October fall day.

While stopping in the local bike shop in Stowe, Vermont, Ed purchased a brand of peanut butter manufactured by a local retailer, one that Rachel had eaten before, and put it in the car for later.

We all rented bikes and started casually and joyfully riding down the bike path. After a while, Rachel was tired, so we decided to split up. I took Rachel back to the shop to return our bikes, and Ed continued on his ride with our younger daughter.

Rachel was hungry, so I gave her a whopping spoonful of the peanut butter Ed had bought in the bike shop. I didn't think twice as she had eaten this local brand before and she was no longer allergic to peanut butter. "Mommy, I don't feel well," Rachel suddenly blurted.

"What's the matter?"

"My tongue is itchy."

Oh No!

I read the label on the peanut butter. The last ingredient in this particular flavor was "Whey Protein Isolate," a milk derivative ingredient commonly used to fortify the protein in bars, beverages, cereals and other food products. "Who puts whey in peanut butter?!" I thought. And for good reason as I would learn later when Rachel was well into her allergy program. Protein isolates change protein into a difficult to digest form and turned out to be Rachel's nemesis. Even when no longer reacting to that which she was most allergic to, she would continue to have difficulty processing anything with whey protein isolate. But at this time, I knew none of this.

I found the backpack in the front of the car with the antihistamine and immediately gave her some. It's a good thing that she stayed with me when we split up because I don't think Ed would have known where the Benadryl and EpiPen were.

The nearest urgent care was just down the road. I drove the car there, but they were closed because it was Sunday.

Oh No! I called 911. "Where's the nearest emergency room?" The police officer told me to stay where I was. He said I would lose my cell phone connection and he wouldn't be able to find me. So I stayed where I was, which happened to be in the parking lot of a real estate office. He sent an ambulance to us and Rachel was observed by the paramedics on a stretcher in the ambulance. A phone call with the doctors at the emergency department determined it was unnecessary to admit her.

Still holding the EpiPen in my hand, the paramedics reassured me that she only had a mild reaction and informed me that I handled it well. Still, I couldn't stop thinking about how bad the allergic reaction could have been. After 45 minutes Rachel was released from the ambulance, walked out of the vehicle and vomited in the parking lot of the real estate office.

While Rachel was still in the ambulance, the police officer drove back to the bike rental place in Stowe to find Ed, my younger daughter and explain why I ran off with Rachel and the car.

We were never charged for the ambulance visit nor did we ever have a chance to thank the paramedics or the police officer for their help.

RACHEL CARRIES HER OWN EPIPEN:
LATE FALL 2012

This incident devastated me. I realized that I could never take food ingredients for granted. Even if I was familiar with the product and it had been deemed safe for Rachel, I *always* had to read the label – especially since I was now a Food Allergy Coach. I also needed Rachel to start taking personal responsibility. What if this had happened and Ed and I weren't there?

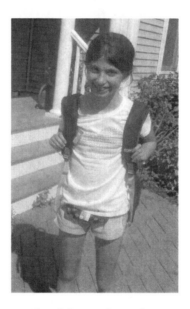

My career coach told me about her granddaughter's friend who carried a little pouch with her so her meds were at hand should she ever need them.

It was time for Rachel to carry her own EpiPen and antihistamine. This way it wouldn't matter if Ed was with her or any other adult.

Online I found a perfect solution: an "EpiBelt." It looked like a fanny pack, just large enough for some of the individually-dosed packages of liquid antihistamine and an EpiPen. Rachel chose her very own black and hot pink polka dot style, and we were in business! Of course I also continued to carry my own survival kit with me. Soon after I started my "Your Food Allergy Coach" business, I trained Rachel how to use the EpiPen by practicing on an orange.

LUNA BAR INCIDENT: MARCH 2013

By this time, I was an expert at label reading. And luckily so. After Rachel outgrew her nut allergy, her diet expanded to include Luna bars containing nuts. We read the label on the Chocolate Peppermint Stick box which said "may contain traces of dairy." Rachel seemed to tolerate these quite well.

And then, one day, we bought a box of the same exact flavor that stated "contains traces of dairy" instead of "may" contain dairy. This minor detail turned out to be a major oversight as Rachel ate part of one and had a mild allergic reaction. We failed to read the label because we had established trust with the many boxes we had bought in the past.

I was irate. How can you have the same product and same flavor with two different allergy cautions? After all, though I read every label thoroughly, it was realistically impossible to do so every time for a product that was trusted. Rachel had eaten hundreds of these bars without any issues.

I sent the company a letter. The customer service department responded by writing that they had followed all FDA guidelines and would notify their "food safety and quality assurance team."

I wrote back. Here's an excerpt.

"Dear Customer Service Department,

I understand that your company followed all FDA guidelines. My concern is the inconsistencies on the labeling of the exact same product. One box of Chocolate Peppermint Stick Luna Bar's is labeled "may contain" and another is labeled "contains" traces of dairy. Why are the products and therefore labels different? Are they made in different factories? Are they made on the same equipment as other bars which contain dairy?

They wrote back to say, while LUNA's recipe has not changed, one of their non-dairy/non-milk ingredients was sourced from a supplier that produces dairy/milk products using the same manufacturing equipment. This was why they changed their labeling allergen statement from **"may contain"** to **"contains"** traces of dairy.

TOFUTTI FUDGE BAR INCIDENT: SEPTEMBER 2013

After this incident, I vowed to never let another morsel of food into Rachel's mouth without reading the label thoroughly. But of course this is not always realistic and there was another incident.

We were in Pittsburgh at Ed's parents' house having a family dinner. Ed's mother made a brisket and we had a lovely dinner. My mother-in-law purposely bought a dairy-free chocolate-fudge Tofutti treat for Rachel to eat for dessert.

Shortly after she ate her treat, she went into the den. As I walked past the den to use the bathroom, I found Rachel sitting on the easy chair. She said she didn't feel well. Her eyes were swollen, she was sneezing, and she had a stomach ache. I immediately whipped out the Benadryl. I was upset as I had no idea why this would be happening. I had checked all the ingredients myself and Tofutti was dairy-free.

After we got home, I wrote Tofutti a letter trying to get to the bottom of the mystery. They wrote me back that there are no eggs, dairy, mustard, or kamut in any of their frozen dessert products. But the product does contain Nutrasweet and sorbitol, artificial sugar substitutes and they suggested that these may have caused the problem.

Or it may have been the cocoa, the bean from which chocolate is made. Because there had been an ongoing world-wide shortage of cocoa, they were now using parts of the cocoa bean they formerly did not use and processing the bean with more alkali. They thought the alkali could cause a reaction, albeit a minor one. As it turned out, Rachel had been sensitive to other chocolate flavors in the past and so it may have been the cocoa bean with more alkali.

Interestingly Rachel intuitively knew not to eat the chocolate Tofutti "cuties" and preferred the vanilla ones. Amazing isn't it how the body knows! A lesson for all of us; listen to your body!

Rachel knew how to read labels and would normally try new things, but these incidents now made her feel a little sketchy about eating new foods. They made the rest of our family nervous as well. Iris was attuned to her sister's reactions and was very cautious and considerate every time there was a potential new issue. As for me, since these incidents happened when we were travelling, I wrote blog posts such as "Traveling to your Vacation Destination" and "Summer Vacation" to help other parents who were in the same situation know they were not alone.

CHAPTER 11

Light at the End
of the Tunnel

It had been months since Rachel last had an allergic reaction. We were living a normal, happy lifestyle in spite of her food allergies. My food allergy coaching business was doing well. I was working with a few clients, sharing practical solutions and teaching workshops to educate others on how to keep their children safe, and empowering them to communicate with others in a positive manner. "I like how you are on top of the issues, but your daughter still does everything and lives a normal life," one client commented.

Yet I was still frustrated.

Having food allergies could be debilitating, not just medically but emotionally. For all of us parents, the social aspect of food allergies was a hassle. Life revolves around food, and having to manage food allergies in almost any group or family situation puts restrictions on everyday life and reduces confidence.

Furthermore, safety concerns still lingered. Though I felt Rachel *should* be safe as long as I knew the ingredients in each product, I never knew with absolute certainty, as I had learned with the *Tofutti* incident and other products Rachel had ingested. One of my client's sons had an allergic reaction to an aged cheddar mac-n-cheese. Her son had eaten cheddar many times without any trouble; the only ingredient that was different on the aged cheddar label was annatto, a natural food coloring. Although her son's doctor denied that he was allergic to annatto, after doing research we discovered that annatto comes from the seed of the achiote tree and that her son could most definitely have an allergic reaction to something coming from a tree.

I wanted more than just to manage the allergies for myself and my clients. I wanted them gone! I didn't want to have to teach other parents about avoiding foods their kids were allergic to or speak with the restaurant manager every time we ate out. Nor did I want to have to worry that Rachel might accidentally eat something she was allergic to when she was out in the real world or visiting a friend.

I became an information hound. Knowledge was power, and power was an enabler.

HOW USEFUL IS ALLERGY TESTING?

On Monday March 18, 2013, I attended a public meeting entitled "Ask the Allergist." Curt Moody, MD, the allergist who spoke, mentioned there were three medically related testing result scenarios:

- Clinically irrelevant positive: the person is eating peanut every day and still tests positive to the allergen in question.
- Clinically relevant positive: the person tests positive in a medical setting and in addition reacts in the real world to the allergen.
- Unknown: the person has never eaten it.

The physician said that false positives outnumbered the real ones 40% of the time and were *hardly ever clinically relevant*. How useful was allergy testing, I wondered?

VERY HELPFUL LECTURE

On April 22, 2013, I attended another fascinating lecture entitled "Changing Concepts in Food Allergy" given by a local Boston allergist, Michael Young, MD and I learned a great deal.

In talking about the inaccuracy of allergy testing, Dr. Young commented on how skin prick or serum testing to related foods may be positive in many cases where the food may be tolerated.

Were people unnecessarily avoiding foods to which they were potentially not allergic?

COMPLETE AVOIDANCE

Dr. Young spoke of the medical communities' focus on complete avoidance of allergens as the only safe treatment. As stated by the Expert Panel of the *Guidelines for the Diagnosis and Management of Food Allergy in the United States: Report of the NIAID* (National Institutes of Health and Infectious Diseases), "allergen avoidance is currently the safest strategy for managing FA."

There is, however, noted Dr. Young, no evidence that strict food avoidance has any effect on the rate of natural remission to a specific food allergen. He mentioned certain case reports discussing how, after the respective foods were avoided the patient experienced a loss of tolerance, and allergies actually worsened.

country	% allergic	told to avoid or feed
USA	25	avoid
UK	69	avoid
Israel	2.1	feed
Philippines	0	feed

Personal notes from the lecture

And he talked about the LEAP study: "Randomized Trial of Peanut Consumption in Infants at Risk for Peanut Allergy," published Feb. 26, 2015 in *The New England Journal of Medicine*. The study stated that Jewish children in Israel were consuming peanut-based products at 7 months of age with very low prevalence to peanut allergy, whereas Jewish children in the United Kingdom, who did not typically consume peanut-based foods in the first year of life, had a much higher incidence of food allergy. The study then hypothesized that early introduction might offer protection from developing that allergen.

DESENSITIZATION TO MILK

Dr. Young also talked about a 2004 study in which there was a successful desensitization to milk and that "dietary inclusion of extensively heated milk and egg protein can expedite development." Yet he cautioned several negatives to the study. For one, patients needed to eat the food every day of their lives or they would lose the desensitization tolerance. And second, being sick with a fever may increase the chances of anaphylaxis.

He talked also about how kids were now outgrowing milk and egg allergy in their teens, compared to 20 years ago when the norm to outgrow milk and egg allergies was typically age 3-5. Could stricter avoidance have caused this, he pondered? I had the very same question.

Interestingly, he also spoke about the problem of avoidance in mother's breastmilk. He said some research was starting to show that early consumption was actually associated with *less* allergy.

After this very informative lecture I wondered if all the avoidance we were told to do was wrong. So many unanswered questions; I had to find a way to get rid of these allergies! There had to be a better way!

And then suddenly the opportunity presented itself to test out calculated exposure rather than complete avoidance.

ENTER ALEXIS

My friend Melissa told me about her cousin Alexis: a naturopath, professional nutritionist, health coach and advanced level practitioner of an allergy elimination technique similar to NAET, which I spoke of earlier. As you may recall, NAET focuses on building and strengthening the body's immune system through energy medicine and other techniques to erase the nervous system's previous reaction and re-imprint a new healthy response. Over several years, Alexis had developed an integrative method of systematic desensitization, a cross between advanced energy medicine and Western technology. Like NAET, it focuses on building and strengthening the body's immune system.

Protocol begins with using an electro-dermal device to evaluate what systems are out of balance or blocked. An Eastern approach, the device is based on the premise that every object has a frequency and the frequency of a particular organism or allergen affects your energy field.

Alexis does a detailed analysis of the health of the gut, as 70% of the immune system is located in the digestive tract. The evaluation looks for bacteria, viruses, candida, mold or parasites that create imbalances in the gut. Further, the evaluation looks at possible side effects from heavy metals or vaccinations that cause an imbalance in the immune system. Next Alexis looks for the presence of mold, dust, additives, chemicals and sweeteners, as these can lock in other allergens and contribute to reactivity.

After the immune system lines up with this special technique, determined by the electro-dermal device, Alexis clears food allergies through systematic desensitization (SD). Similar to how phobias are healed, systematic desensitization, a Western concept introduces the allergen in tolerable, minute doses and increases the dosage to build tolerance to the allergen.

WOULD RACHEL GO FOR IT?

Could Alexis' technique of marrying Western (systematic desensitization) and Eastern (energy medicine) concepts reprogram Rachel's nervous system to stop her from reacting to her allergies? I felt very hopeful. Now I had to find out how Rachel felt about it.

So, the next day, while we were driving home I said, "Rachel, I think I found someone who can help you get rid of your allergies. Would you be interested in trying something new?"

"Mom, I would do ANYTHING to get rid of my allergies," and then she added, "Well almost anything. I wouldn't cut off my arm."

Gotta love that kid!

I was proud of my daughter for understanding all the information I had learned and shared with her about food allergies. I was also excited because she was willing to try something new. We would definitely pursue this new method!

Using the contact request form found on Alexis's website, I requested an appointment. Her office called to inform me that clients were waiting *an average of 3 years* to see Alexis once they were placed on the waitlist. "Please put us on the waitlist," I uttered.

In the meantime, we began to visualize what our life would be like without the food allergies – both medically and without all the social barriers!

GROUNDBREAKING ARTICLE
While waiting, I educated myself as much as I could about different approaches to clear food allergies. An important *New York Times Magazine* Article, "The Allergy Buster: Can a Radical New Treatment Save Children With Severe Food Allergies" published on March 7, 2013, discussed a clinical trial by Dr. Kari Nadeau, an associate professor of allergies and immunology at Stanford University School of Medicine and Lucile Packard Children's Hospital. The article described the success Dr. Nadeau and others were having using oral immunotherapy to desensitize children with severe peanut allergies. As the article states, "The treatment re-educated the hyperactive immune systems of allergy patients by giving them minute doses of peanut every day, gradually escalating the amount over the course of

several years. Eventually patients build up their tolerance for the food, and it is no longer dangerous."

The concept was not new. As the article went on to
state,

> "The therapy has been used successfully for envi-
> ronmental allergies for decades, by giving patients
> small injections of pollen or cat dander or other aller-
> gens, but it was considered too dangerous to try with
> food allergies until recently. A study testing various
> allergens was pioneered in Europe in the 1980s, and
> in the past five years, ongoing studies at Mount Si-
> nai School of Medicine in New York and other centers
> have shown that children can be safely desensitized to
> a single allergen, peanut, and, in separate trials, to
> milk and egg."

Milk and egg! Rachel's worst triggers!

ALLERGY CONFERENCE

On November 5, 2014, I attended a restaurant conference at the Seaport Hotel in Boston that catered to
the allergy community. One of the speakers was Ming
Tsai. Ming's son had once been allergic to seven out of
the eight most common food allergens and was no longer allergic. Alexis had brought his son through a five-
year process and eliminated his food allergies. To Ming
it was extraordinary that his family had actually gone
on a trip to China the previous summer: "You can't go
to China with a peanut allergy because everything is
cooked in peanut oil."

Everything he said reinforced my reasoning for wanting to work with Alexis. Now we just needed to wait our turn.

ALLERGIST APPOINTMENT: OCTOBER, 2013

It was time to check in with Rachel's allergist because I wanted to discuss with her all of the issues we were having, especially the Luna bar and Tofutti incidents. So in October of 2013 I made an appointment.

I brought with us the Trader Joe's cereal bars that contained a small amount of dairy (somehow Rachel was able to tolerate these bars) and asked the allergist if my daughter could eat one in her office. She was appalled. After skin testing, the allergist said our daughter's allergies were getting worse! She strongly suggested that we avoid all she was allergic to, including eggs, dairy and mustard.

I mentioned the New York Times magazine article and the work Dr. Nadeau was doing with oral immunotherapy. Again, she was appalled, stating that the information in the article was inaccurate and that certain important details were omitted. She sternly warned us to vigilantly avoid the foods that Rachel was allergic to and to read labels more diligently.

This comment took me by surprise. As a food allergy coach, I was doing training on label reading and was well aware of how to read a label for Rachel's allergens. The issue wasn't parenting or label reading. The exposures Rachel had were accidental and the reactions were inconsistent.

As I walked out of her office, I became even more baffled, wondering how one doctor could lecture about tolerance while another continued to give advice about avoidance. How could one doctor publish an article in the prestigious New York Times Magazine about cutting-edge research when my local doctor was appalled at the new research and concerned for our daughter's safety?

I became more and more convinced that Alexis' thinking outside of the box would heal Rachel of her allergies.

A week later I received a copy of a letter that the allergist had sent to Rachel's pediatrician which, in addition to stating all of which Rachel was allergic also stated,

"I am very concerned about the number of reactions Rachel has had over the number of years that I have followed her which far surpass any other child I follow. She continues to eat products with advisory labeling, despite the fact that she has reacted to such products. We know that not every item with advisory labeling has the same level of contamination, but clearly occasionally these items have a large enough amount to trigger a reaction. I discussed with her mother that all products with advisory labeling should be avoided. I reviewed again with her mother that a number of studies have shown that the level of cross

*contamination is the same across the board regard-
less of the type of labeling. In addition, the frequency
of contamination with milk is much higher than for
peanut...the rate of contamination can exceed 80% for
chocolate products with advisory labeling."*

The tone of this letter distressed me. I felt as if she
were accusing me of being negligent with my daughter, that, in spite of the extreme caution I took with everything Rachel ate and extreme diligence in reading
labels she was blaming me for the severity of Rachel's
food allergies.

On top of that, while she had done an excellent job
documenting her findings and our conversation from
Rachel's appointment, I did not feel as if she had been
especially helpful. I needed answers. How could we get
this help and where could we find it? If she typified conventional medicine, I needed to look elsewhere.

True, modern medicine has done wonders for our
society; we have penicillin and open heart surgery, for
example. My daughter's bilateral reinsertion cured her
hydronephrosis. I was treated for pre-eclampsia after
my second daughter was born, and I had an emergency
appendectomy which probably saved my life. Yet clearly
Western medicine had not yet fully understood food allergies; it looked like strict avoidance was not the only
solution. Yet, as the big picture was not yet understood,
many practitioners were not willing to even discuss tolerance and desensitization.

Time to move on.

MORE ENCOURAGING NEWS ABOUT SYSTEMATIC DESENSITIZATION

My confidence in Alexis's treatment was further bolstered as I began to discover other parents who had success with this approach on their kids. For example, my friend Nancy (Chapter 7) whose son had serious digestive constraints had recently been healed by Alexis.

Another note of encouragement came from Tiffany, a friend of Rachel's from her honors chorus program. Tiffany told us of two people she knew who underwent the same allergy elimination process. I contacted each of these moms and I learned encouraging news along with details of their experience. For instance, once someone started systematic desensitization, the resulting numbers during allergy testing increased and almost doubled until the body got used it. But then the numbers eventually declined. That sounded scary. But it was also revealing. That Rachel accidentally ate those Trader Joes cereal bars before she started her program with Alexis might have been why the allergist said her allergies were getting worse.

Within a few months I had spoken with at least five people whose children no longer had food allergies after completing systematic desensitization. Alexis was our silver bullet, our light at the end of the tunnel. We couldn't wait to start her program.

PART THREE
ALLERGY ELIMINATION

CHAPTER 12

Day Finally Arrives

"At first they'll ask you why you did it,
but then they will ask you how you did it."

~Unknown

In December 2013, after being on her waitlist for about two years, Alexis personally called us to schedule our first appointment.

I will now share with you part of my actual diary during Rachel's therapy that includes the foods she ate and the order in which she started eating them. There is, however a caveat. To respect this special desensitization process and to discourage anyone reading this book from trying desensitization on their own, I will not give the exact progression of measurements or specific details of the process. I am describing our experience for informational purposes only and sternly warn against any self-treatment as this would be dangerous! This process is emotional, detail-oriented and highly calculated. It can only be done after the immune system is in proper balance. As such, it must be done *only* under the guidance, support, and coaching from a properly trained Certified Health Coach or advanced practitioner in good standing with the method. Each person undergoing desensitization must have an individualized plan set up by the trained practitioner.

This was Rachel's plan.

FOOD DIARY, PART 1
INITIAL APPOINTMENT: JANUARY 4, 2014
Our first meeting with Alexis was a scheduled two-hour appointment on a Saturday. We were told to bring our last allergy testing results, plus I brought the last letter we received from the allergist.

FIRST STEPS
Alexis began by using the electro-dermal device to evaluate Rachel's system. She found that she needed to work on ridding Rachel of allergies to mold, dust, refined, and unrefined sugar. She also needed to work on the chemicals Rachel was exposed to in her everyday life, such as cleaning products, personal care products like shampoo and toothpaste, cat and dog dander, and birch tree pollen to eliminate cross reactivity. Further, she would work on heavy metals as Rachel had recently started wearing metal braces and this could impact her immune system.

WHAT TO EAT
Together, we devised a clear plan to enable Rachel to safely eat the things to which she was allergic. The technique would require my daughter to eat every day, in specified small increasing amounts the foods she had for so long been instructed not to eat. This was done

over time to encourage food tolerance and cause the least amount of processing possible.

Most times Rachel didn't react at all to the changes in her diet. For her it was just eating as a normal kid. This was life, and in life, nothing is ever perfect, foolproof, or certain.

Nevertheless, some processing would be inevitable.

Rachel, however was a real trooper. She knew that to be able to eat the foods that her friends were eating, including pizza and ice cream, cookies with butter and cupcakes with buttercream she might have to go through some discomfort as her body adjusted to the introduction of even the most miniscule amounts of the food to which she was allergic.

But as long as we didn't "cut off her arm," she was game. This was going to change all of our lives for the better.

HELPFUL SUPPLEMENTS
In addition to the foods Rachel was to eat, she also had to take daily a specific type of probiotic to promote the growth of beneficial microorganisms in the intestines and to support the upper and lower intestinal tracts. This particular probiotic also contained a prebiotic for even more growth of beneficial microorganisms in the intestines. We also brought with us each week a bottle of plain water which Alexis would put on her electro-dermal device. Rachel would take drops of

this water on a daily basis. It was specific to whatever we were working on each week. We were also told to buy Alka Seltzer Gold as it alkalizes the gut and puts the body in balance. "Alka" became our best friend.

LOGISTICS

This process was a huge commitment requiring regular weekly office visits, daily assignments and accountability to these assignments. No worries. Feeling blessed to have these appointments after a two-year wait, we willingly and gratefully dedicated one day per week after school to commute to and from Alexis's office for our weekly half-hour appointments.

At home, we followed daily, detailed instructions. I blocked off more than an hour each day to measure and calmly be with Rachel during the time she would eat her new foods. I ensured she was relaxed, as excitement increased heart rate and breathing and could have an unfavorable effect. The "mind/body" connection was a very important component in the overall desensitization process.

TIMELINE

Based on my prior research with other parents whose children had completed this process, I surmised that it could take about two and a half years to complete. Alexis suggested that we initially make a commitment of one year to the program. This was not a problem. Rachel and I were willing to dedicate any amount of time necessary to get rid of her allergies.

2-27-14

This was our first week of desensitization. Since our daughter had trouble in the past with chocolate processed with alkali, Alexis worked on this with her electro dermal device. It was almost like training for the big leagues – egg, dairy and mustard – except using nonpareil chocolate, not milk chocolate. We would save that for later on in the therapy. Rachel was thrilled! Imagine being told part of your therapy after your immune system was balanced is to eat chocolate. It sounded like a reward.

After Rachel started eating a tiny bit of the nonpareil, we worked up over a period of time to a serving. Nothing unpleasant happened!

Seven weeks into her therapy, she started eating a pure dark chocolate nonpareil that was processed with alkali.

We were ready to move on to the next allergen and Alexis told me to bring something with kamut the following week.

EMOTIONS AND GRATITUDE

Emotions play a powerful role in the strength of the immune system, something research into the psychology of the mind/body connection has well documented. For this reason, Alexis asked Rachel to come up with a mantra, a phrase repeated to aid concentration in meditation. This would help her cope with any fears that might come up during therapy.

While repeating this mantra, Alexis told her to tap on specific meridian points, a technique called EFT or Emotional Freedom Technique. Tapping with your fingertips stimulates meridian points and literally taps into your body's own energy and healing power. EFT has been successfully shown to not only help emotionally but to eliminate fears and phobias.

In addition, Rachel was asked to keep a *grateful journal* and to write down daily three things for which she was grateful. Initially she wrote down what she was grateful for in her little red notebook, but eventually she would just tell me instead. They were little things like what she did with her friends or when school was cancelled because of a snowy day.

She was especially grateful for getting a new Kindle as she was a voracious reader. One time, after Ed put her allowance on her Kindle, she announced, "Those are the two things a girl needs: money and a book." Reading proved to be one of the important things that would keep her mind calm and distracted on this life-changing journey.

3-6-14

Alexis continued to work on mustard, dairy, whey, lactose, casein, and eggs with her electro-dermal screening device. Rachel's immune system was not yet in balance for these food substances, but she was improving.

To ready her for the big step of clearing her of her major allergies, Alexis asked Rachel to decide what major allergens she wanted to work on first. Rachel decided to start with egg. Alexis told her to come up with a list of foods that contained egg that she wanted to try to eat.

After egg, Rachel would tackle dairy. Dairy was a bit more difficult since it contains more complex proteins. Finally Rachel would complete the program with mustard.

To further the mind/body connection, Alexis told Rachel to create a vision board and to hang it on her bedroom wall as a constant reminder of her goals; visualizing what her life would be like once she achieved her goals would make it easier for her to achieve them.

She was also asked to make a list of how her life would change when she didn't have allergies anymore. To further help motivate her, Rachel was asked to create a reward for each goal she would achieve. For achieving her egg goal, she decided she would have breakfast in bed. For achieving her dairy goal, she envisioned eating a giant piece of cheesecake, a desire likely gotten from me. When I was nursing and told to avoid dairy because Rachel was allergic, I craved a big giant piece of cheesecake –my love of cheesecake was no secret in our family. Later on, pizza and ice cream would become Rachel's favorite foods and cheesecake would lose its excitement.

In the meantime, we were still working on the chocolate at home. Rachel's kamut was in balance, so we started working on it simultaneously with the chocolate by increasing it in small amounts.

5-1-14
Four months after our first weekly appointment, we achieved an important milestone: Rachel's immune system was in balance and the awaited allergy protocol could begin.

As Rachel had desired, we started working on the desensitization process for egg. In the next office visit, we brought in a chopped up hard-boiled egg. Alexis put a minutely small piece of the egg on Rachel's lip. It was practically invisible! I was confident that nothing would happen because I trusted the process and we had no trouble with the kamut or chocolate processed with alkali.

Nothing did happen.

Still, watching Rachel purposely come into direct contact with something that in the past had made her so sick sent chills down my spine. Even though it was such a small amount, I thought about the egg pasta she had unintentionally eaten at overnight camp and reminded myself how far we had come.

Alexis gave us very specific instructions to follow for the week to desensitize the egg. Rachel was to eat the egg in the morning before she went to school. I had to measure the amount she would put in her mouth each morning. This presented a bit of a challenge for me as mornings were already a busy time for our family.

We did this religiously every morning, gradually increasing the amount of egg Rachel ate according to a projected egg measurement assignment. All was written down carefully in a notebook that I checked off daily according to Alexis' instructions. In this way, we should meet Rachel's goal of eating baked-in egg at the four-week overnight camp she would attend that summer.

The first time I purchased half a dozen eggs was completely life changing. We *never* had eggs in the house. And now we were allowed to have eggs in the house and we were continuously eating them. Amazing!

Excitedly, I started thinking about cooking with baked-in egg, something our whole family could now enjoy. What products would Rachel like to eat? I decided to bake a batch of Trader Joes muffin mix that we had always used with Ener-G egg replacer. Using a single mini bread mold and a cupcake mold, I made a baker's dozen -- with eggs!

Rachel loved the muffin, her first food with baked-in egg. She also started eating egg noodles, as well as brownies and cupcakes that contained egg. At first, she was timid about putting these products in her mouth, but once she tasted them, she really liked them and wanted more!

As for me, my job was to make sure she ate only the specified amount for that day.

6-9-14
We were told to buy matzo balls. Matzo balls have eggs in them, and now Rachel, like everyone else could have them in her chicken soup. This was so important. Chicken soup with matzo balls is a Jewish traditional food. She was so excited!

I went to a kosher, dairy-free bakery and purchased a bag of six challah rolls, made with egg, and some frozen matzo balls. The owner told me how many eggs were in a batch of challah rolls, and we calculated the amount of egg per matzo ball. To keep Rachel safe, we used this measurement information to determine how much egg Rachel was eating. In this way, I could give her a challah roll and matzo ball gradually in increasing amounts.

I was grateful that Rachel was able to eat the egg, not only to heal her allergies but also because egg provided her with some protein to give her more energy in the morning. Imagine the nutrients her body was getting.

6-12-14
On this day, Rachel had a bump on her lip indicating a little "processing.'" To be extra careful, we stayed at the same measurement the next day instead of increasing it.

6-18-14

We were now using large grade A eggs and I measured the number of tablespoons in a hard-boiled egg. We had to realistically determine what our goal was when she went away to camp, and this gave us our answer. If she could eat 4-½ teaspoons, this would be half of an egg. While the measurement for straight egg was exact, the items for baked-in egg were more subjective. So I wrote in my assignment book which items we were to work on which days. This week we were working on the egg noodles or challah roll and either brownie or cupcake.

NOT ALL A PIECE OF CAKE

All this may sound straight forward: just give this to her to eat. In fact, getting it right was challenging in two ways. First Rachel had to agree to which item she would eat on which day – remember the importance of the mind/body connection. Once I knew her choice, we then had many discussions over the details of portion sizes and the rotation of different foods. One minor challenge was her over-eagerness to try these new foods. I had to limit her from eating more egg than she was ever able to eat before.

Second, it was a challenge to find the time in the day to work on all these new foods as we had to space out the timing of introducing and measuring these new foods with her meals to isolate any issues. We obviously had more time on the weekends when she didn't have school, but we still needed to keep up with our daily regimen.

Yet these challenges were minor. What was important was that she was building tolerance so we no longer had to worry about accidental exposure to egg due to cross contact and a potential allergic reaction. Things were going well. We knew we made the right choice in starting this procedure!

CHAPTER 13

Summer Camp 2014

My daughters were getting ready to go to overnight camp for 28 days. We were all excited. Being with her friends was an important part of Rachel's mental and emotional well-being and a reward for her hard work.

To maintain tolerance, our plan was to stay with the same measured amount of egg for the entire month she would be at camp. And the camp was cooperative, giving us confidence that Rachel would be OK. Though we would not make progress, we would not lose momentum.

And then, a snag. On June 24, four days before my daughters would leave for camp, Rachel made an announcement. "I hate eating egg." Oh no! We reminded her that she must eat egg. If she stopped the process, she would lose all the progress she made and not be able to eat egg in the things she enjoyed like the other kids.

Our little trooper understood. We just had to figure out how to make the egg more palatable. Tornado dust to the rescue. Tornado dust is the topping of an "everything" bagel – onion, garlic, sesame, poppy, and salt. By dipping her half of a hard-boiled egg in this topping, she was able to tolerate the taste for the remaining four mornings before she left for camp.

INSTRUCTIONS TO KEEP RACHEL SAFE

Rachel was doing her part to prepare herself for a safe experience at camp and I had to do mine.

Full Report

The first thing I did was to send the camp director a full report on Rachel's allergies: what she was allergic to; the signs of a potential allergic reaction; what to do in case of an allergic reaction. I explained the egg therapy she was undergoing and that Rachel would eat half of an egg for breakfast every morning and some baked-in products containing eggs every day that I would provide. They would freeze them, and she would eat them each day as I requested.

I printed several copies of a final letter of instruction to give to the counselor, health center, chef, and director so that everyone would be on the same page.

Alerting the Chef

This camp had a special chef in charge of all campers and staff who knew how to handle kids with special dietary needs. That allayed my anxiety. But I still felt the need to speak to the chef and it was a good thing I

FROM ANAPHYLAXIS TO BUTTERCREAM

did. While the director alerted the counselors and nursing staff about Rachel's allergies and special needs, she omitted (not intentionally I'm sure) alerting the chef, who was unaware of the whole allergy elimination procedure. I gave the chef a printed list of instructions along with all of the baked-in items Rachel would need throughout the month and he put these items in the freezer.

The camp also gave Rachel free rein to go into the kitchen before every meal to discuss with the chef what foods she could and could not eat. If the planned meals had nothing she or any of the other kids with special dietary needs could eat, he would make a special meal for them.

Nursing Staff
Next, I gave the nursing staff all of the items listed on the instruction sheet.

We informed them that Rachel carries an "EpiBelt" with her at all times containing one auto injector and Benadryl, but that she has never injected epinephrine into her own leg and is too young to be expected to take responsibility on her own. In case of an emergency, the nurse would have to inject the medicine.

The health staff was well informed, ready for us and happy to accommodate. In fact, the whole camp was wonderful about complying with our unusual requests, and they followed all our instructions. Prior to drop off, we were told the director took one of Rachel's bunk counselors aside and said "I need you to be on top of Rachel and her allergies." We were grateful and more at ease.

LOSS OF COMMUNICATION

Yet, I was still nervous that all would run smoothly, made worse by a strict rule of the camp: phone calls to and from parents were not allowed because they could cause "moments of sadness" or "homesickness." Rachel *would* be allowed to speak with her health coach twice during the four week period, but she *would not* be permitted to talk with me at all! This exception was made for medical purposes as part of her therapy.

Of course the camp nurse or director could call me at any time if there was an issue. I could also call the health center or email the chef.

Still, my direct communication with her was cut off and that was hard for me. The kids were completely unplugged without texting devices or phones – smart camp! We could of course send letters through the U.S. mail or the camp's e-letter system.

7-2-14

I received a disturbing letter from Rachel. The environment at an overnight camp is full of dust, mold, dirt, farm animals, pool water, bugs, grass, tree pollen, and lots of kids in a crowded bunk. These factors were affecting her. She wrote, "Dear Mom, today I might have had an allergic reaction to the paper maché a.k.a.

(grass, paper, sticky notes + water) Love you! Rachel."
Heart, smiley face, peace sign pictures.

What did this "allergic reaction" mean? I needed to
be able to speak directly with my daughter to know exactly what she was talking about but rules are rules and
I couldn't. This was incredibly hard for me, but if something was really wrong, the nurse would have called.

She didn't, so I should have been reassured. But as
a mother, I couldn't stop thinking and worrying about
what was going on at camp.

7-3-14
Her next letter was profoundly disturbing, *"Allergic
reactions every day."*

We tried to keep in mind that kids live in the mo-
ment and that what happens during the time they send
a letter may not be what is happening when we receive
the letter. Still, I worried.

7-7-14
The camp nurse called me to tell me she had to give
Rachel some antihistamine (Benadryl) and wanted to
know if we could put her on anything stronger. I suggested Zyrtec for the remainder of the month at camp
to be given in the morning. The nurse agreed. Rachel
had not been on Zyrtec in months, but she was on it
the previous year at camp. The nurse also mentioned
Rachel's other visits to the health center, which now explained her letter stating "allergic reactions every day."

The nurse put Rachel's letter into perspective.

July 1st: a bug bite. They gave her Benadryl. Also July 1st: About 6 hives on each arm from the sticky stuff. July 4th: Something else during the carnival.

Another time she was congested. Her reactions sounded like they were environmental, not food related. Sigh of relief.

Rachel was in the room when the nurse called. Though I was not allowed to speak with her, she reassured me that overall, Rachel was doing well. She was eating half of a hard-boiled egg every morning.

The nurse said Rachel looked happy and was chatting with another kid. I may have been a wreck but my dear daughter had more important things to do than to worry about her health! My daughter is such an amazing, resilient child!

Outside of these few allergy-related letters, I received great letters from her. She was happy at camp and in spite of the initial scare, we met our desensitization goals without any processing.

CHAPTER 14

Achieving New Milestones:
Food Diary, Part 2

MILESTONE: JULY 30, 2014:
Rachel started eating French toast!

She liked eating anything with baked-in egg, but refused to eat anything with straight egg. "I hate the way it tastes." I worried that her preferences might affect her tolerance to egg. If she stopped eating it, what would happen in the future if she decided to eat something that had more than one egg in it? Would she be able to tolerate it?

And I wondered why she started disliking straight egg after reaching so many wonderful milestones. Was it the taste, texture or perhaps both? Or perhaps she didn't like it because she was still allergic and her body reacted negatively. I wondered how many people didn't like eating something because of an allergy issue.

Still, I felt she had to eat straight egg. I tried to make her things that contained straight egg, like an omelet, but to no avail; she wouldn't eat it. She did however continue to eat baked goods and other things that contained egg.

ORGANIC FOOD

Until this time, I hadn't given much thought as to whether a food was organic or not. But as I was becoming more and more educated as to what constitutes healthy eating, I now understood the importance of eating organic food. Organic food is grown without the pesticides, herbicides, antibiotics and hormones in commercial food, as well as other harmful substances and is therefore far healthier. Many research studies have discovered a relationship between these substances in our food supply and disease like heart disease, Alzheimers, autoimmune disorders, chronic diseases and cancer.

As a result, we used only foods with organic ingredients when introducing any new foods. This allowed Rachel's body to get used to the previous allergens better than before we introduced any processed foods.

9-5-14

The month of September was our most momentous milestone. We started working on dairy! Alexis told us to purchase either Plain or French Vanilla Fat Free Stonyfield yogurt in the white and blue container.

As we were still having trouble getting Rachel to eat egg, Alexis suggested giving her something exciting that she enjoyed containing straight egg. Some examples were custard made with almond milk, meringue cookies that were sold at Trader Joe's and Whole Foods, Martha Stewart wedding cake frosting on vegan cupcakes, waffles, key lime pie, and the Belle and Evans Gluten Free chicken nuggets that have egg in the coating. But the more I tried, the more our mother/preteen power struggles increased with resistance. I was unsuccessful in getting her to eat most of these foods and relented.

10-23-14
Once Rachel started middle school she needed to leave the house by 7:10 a.m. This meant we had to shift our schedule to an earlier time so she could consume her carefully measured daily allotment of organic fat free yogurt around 6:30 a.m. Super early for us, it was a big adjustment and left us little time to eat both egg and dairy before she had to leave for school. We needed time in between, so sometimes we did one before school and one after school.

And then there was the problem of how to get her to eat straight egg as in an egg omelet, egg salad sandwich (with mayo), or pancakes three times a week, which she needed to do. As it turned out, daddy's little girl resisted her father less than she resisted her mother and Ed got her to eat egg in the morning. I in turn did the dairy measurement later in the day after she got home from school.

This schedule seemed to work as there was no processing.

11-13-14

We achieved another milestone this week: we gradually started introducing Breyers *Organic* ice cream without egg. All of the other ice cream brands contained too many chemicals.

Imagine. My daughter, who needed epinephrine because she licked a popsicle that contained dairy, was now eating ice cream for breakfast. What a dream for a kid with an anaphylactic dairy allergy!

12-5-14

Another milestone! Rachel brought a package of *Back to Nature* organic cheese crackers with her to school for the first time!

But there was also a scare. At 8:00 p.m., Rachel ate the ice cream and "processed" it: her lips were swollen and she said her stomach hurt. I gave her Alka Seltzer Gold and antihistamine. To help lessen the emotional impact, we did her mantra while doing tapping (EFT).

Apparently, the later in the day she ate something, the more it compromised her immune system. We needed to stick to doing the therapy in the morning.

FIRST YEAR MILESTONE

In December 2014 we reached the "break-even point" in Rachel's desensitization process. We were one year into the program and three months into the dairy process. Rachel was eating more of the things she was once allergic to than we were avoiding. We were thrilled. But this was not a completely linear process. She did have one major and two minor setbacks.

MAJOR PROCESSING INCIDENT: DECEMBER 14, 2014

On this day, the kids went to school two hours later than normal so the teachers could engage in professional development.

Around 6:30 AM, Rachel ate her allotted portion of dairy. Since she had an extra two hours that morning, I decided to make a pumpkin muffin mix. I added an extra egg to try to get more egg in her, so the batter had 3 eggs instead of 2. This turned out to be a bad idea.

At 8:30 a.m., she ate two muffins that I calculated as 43% of an egg. This should have been fine since she was able to eat a whole piece of French toast. But this turned out be another big mistake as apparently either her immune system was compromised or the combination of the two former allergens together caused a major processing incident.

At 9:00 a.m., Rachel said she didn't feel well; she felt itchy. I thought "itchy" meant that her skin was dry and she needed some moisturizing lotion, not allergy processing as there was no sign of any. This was half an hour after she ate anything.

Then her eyes started swelling up. I gave her chewable antihistamine tablets but the allergies soon got worse and I called Alexis.

"I'm really worried. She's covered in hives. Eyes still swollen after antihistamine." I took a picture of her swollen eyes and texted it to her. She called me. After calming me down, as I was close to panic, she expressed concern as she hadn't instructed me to put an extra egg in the muffins.

Given the hives and swelling, I contemplated giving her an EpiPen. But she was breathing fine, and we lived less than a mile from the hospital. Also how would I explain all of this to the hospital staff? And my trust in the drug/medical community was waning. I did however take the EpiPen out as I waited and carefully watched her.

Here's the amazing part...

At 12:45 p.m., she was hungry and went downstairs to eat the lunch that I had packed for her which included:

- ½ tuna sandwich w/mayo (eggs in mayo)
- 2 mini muffins (eggs in muffins)
- 2 clementine oranges
- 1 large bowl of chicken soup with carrots and egg noodles.

I was going to give this to her for dinner, but she was still hungry.

Astonished, I sat across from her at the table watching her eat all of these things. How could this be? If she was still allergic to eggs, wouldn't the processing/reaction have gotten worse?

It didn't. She wanted to eat them, didn't think anything of it, and just moved forward. That's my Rachel!

And then she was still hungry and wanted to eat cheese crackers. Imagine! But I told her to wait a little while.

At 4:00 p.m., the antihistamine had worn off and I did not give her more medicine. Yet she ate the cheese crackers and was fine. Thank goodness! This was the only day during the entire eighteen month process that she was too sick to go to school and one of two days when I had to contemplate giving her epinephrine. Thinking about this day still fills me with panic.

MINOR INCIDENTS IN DECEMBER
A week or so after the major incident, Rachel had two minor processing incidents in the same week. This meant we could not increase the amount of ice cream she was eating every day. And so, to maintain her tolerance, she ate the same amount daily for a month.

TRAVELING A BIT EASIER
In December, we went to a wedding in Philly. Though Rachel was still avoiding dairy (including cheese) when we were out, she ate a specific portion of Breyers organic ice cream in the morning, organic cheese crackers in

the afternoon, and some baked-in products in specific amounts of eggs and dairy at other times during the day.

No processing!

STARTING A NEW YEAR
Egg Status
Last summer Rachel was eating one whole scrambled egg; that meant she should be able to eat straight eggs now. But we were concerned that she may have lost her tolerance as we had discontinued giving her straight egg because she hated it so much. Baked-in eggs were fine, as were baked-in eggs and dairy. As it turned out she went to a hibachi restaurant, ordered egg fried rice which contained one whole egg, and ate all that was on her plate! Go figure.

Eggs and Dairy
At this point, Rachel could eat eggs and dairy together. But we could not give her ice cream too late in the day; the more tired she got, the less well her immune system functioned. As you can see, the whole process can be complicated and requires precise planning and execution – another important reason to never try this at home on your own!

Rachel was now eating dairy three times a day. One of these times was always baked-in, like a small piece of cake or a small amount of butter on toast. I measured these foods and rotated them so she would integrate these foods slowly into her diet, once with the carefully measured allotment of ice cream and a third time per day with a specific number of organic cheese crackers at lunch plus a tuna sandwich with mayo.

Soon after the New Year, we slowly started working on her eating organic mozzarella cheese in small increasing amounts.

Milk Chocolate: January 11
By mid-January, we had reached another milestone: We could start working on milk chocolate. How heavenly was that!

Alexis told us to buy a Hershey's bar because the chocolate rectangles were easy to break and measure. But upon the first tasting, Rachel said it tasted "awful and disgusting." What a dilemma! Almost the entire planet loves Hershey's milk chocolate, but not Rachel. I could not force her to eat it. The solution? Gourmet chocolate!

We bought Rachel some Dolfin cinnamon milk chocolate made in Belgium. Upon tasting a tiny piece, Rachel said, "Yummmm" with a smile and asked for more. Success!

Why would she find the American chocolate disgusting and the European chocolate yummy? European chocolate is made with purer ingredients than chemical-laden popular American chocolate bar.

When your palate speaks, listen. Rachel had a discerning gourmet palate, another one of our amazing daughter's talents.

SCARE AT SCHOOL JANUARY 23, 2015

Rachel normally ate breakfast at 6:30 and walked to school with a friend at 7:10. On this particular morning she was tired. The organic mozzarella cheese stick sat there as she stared at it until 6:45; finally she began to eat it.

At 7:10 she had not yet taken her probiotic – recall that she took a probiotic daily to help her improve her gut health. Announcing that she would take it when she got home, she rushed out the door for school. I wasn't concerned. Not taking the probiotic wouldn't cause an allergic reaction. And, as the parent of an 11-year-old pre-teen, I needed to pick my battles carefully, so I didn't insist that she take it.

My husband left for the gym at this time and drove past Rachel and her friends as they were walking to school. He slowed down to check up on Rachel, offered her a ride and drove her part way with her friends.

When she got to school, her throat was dry and she felt thirsty, an unusual event. She went to her homeroom class, and some 40 minutes later felt unwell. She called me at 7:50 and said her allergies were bothering her. She asked me to bring the probiotic, her "allergy pill" to school. Interesting. Her probiotic was not her allergy pill but somehow Rachel knew her body craved it. Clearly, a mind/body component played out in this incident.

I told her to get the Alka Seltzer Gold from her locker and bring it to the nurse. But the nurse would not let her take the medication because she needed a doctor's permission. At this point I had driven to the school and was just parking the car when the nurse called me on my cell phone. I told her I was in the parking lot and would be there in two seconds.

Rachel's eyes were swollen and her nose was stuffed up and she was blowing it. She had one small hive on her stomach, but nowhere else. The nurse told me she was not allowed to carry medication around with her. Given Rachel's life threatening food allergies, this was of course absurd; but rules are rules as far as the school was concerned!

I immediately gave Rachel Alka Seltzer Gold, but she was still stuffy and her eyes were swollen. If the nurse had given it to her, the processing may have subsided sooner, but instead we lost ten minutes due to a silly protocol that I'm at a loss to explain.

By 8:10 I was still concerned and gave her a chewable antihistamine tablet and the probiotic. The nurse told us that a student "cannot stay in school if she takes an antihistamine because she needs to be observed."

The nurse was concerned about her taking so much medication; Alka Seltzer Gold and antihistamine may be over-the-counter, but they were still medication. I reminded myself that the nurse was just following protocol. Rachel wrote a note to her friend to let her know that they would not be walking home together and I took her home.

By the time we got home, Rachel felt better. I texted Alexis, "Rachel had a full cheese stick. She's OK but was sent home from school."

She called me immediately. As she could hear the panic in my voice – no matter how much experience I had with these "processing" days it was still emotional for me – she talked me off the wall to allay my anxiety. As messages to the brain play a huge part in this process, she reminded me that Rachel had sat there in the morning for 15 minutes and didn't eat the mozzarella cheese. "We want her to be excited about it," she said. "She needs to want it. This makes a huge difference... she's hitting an energetic knot...you could give her the cheese when she gets home from school and the ice cream two hours later."

My panic subsided. I don't know what I would have done if Alexis had not been my rock of Gibraltar during the hard times. Having support from a properly trained practitioner is another important reason why NO ONE should try this process on their own!

In spite of the processing, Rachel was still hungry and ate like a normal kid. I was terrified but she took it in stride and moved on! I am forever amazed at her resiliency!

Throughout the day, I observed what she ate and how she felt.

AT 9:20, she ate guacamole and chips as a snack, nothing to which she was ever allergic. A half hour later, she ate organic baked-in cheese crackers for a snack. Her eyes were still a little swollen, but nothing happened.

By 11:15, her eyes were still a little swollen, but she did not have bags under them like earlier. She was sneezing often and was tired from the antihistamine.

By 12:15, she was still feeling tired, but the antihistamine was wearing off. She ate a tuna sandwich with mayonnaise (egg) for lunch.

I called the nurse at school to see if she could go back to school but the nurse said she needed to wait six hours after taking antihistamine. Protocol was protocol, no exceptions! So Rachel sat on the couch reading a book.

By 2:30, she needed to eat dairy. As we were out of her Breyers Organic ice cream, we went to the supermarket. There Rachel also picked out the organic frozen pizza she would be able to eat once she was able to eat an entire cheese stick without any processing issues, something I had encouraged her to do to capitalize on the power of visualization. If you see it, you will

have the goal imbedded in your brain and think, "I'm
going to have that pizza and I will eventually be able to
have lunch with my friends."

On the way out the door, Rachel said she was hungry and wanted a snack. I suggested some strawberries,
but she asked if she could eat a chocolate chip mixed
salty oats Kayak cookie. These cookies contained butter
and eggs, but Rachel didn't think anything of it.

I wanted to say "no" because she processed that
morning. What if it happened again? But I also wasn't
going to stop her if she really wanted it, so I said, "OK,
but be sure to bring your EpiBelt." Rachel brought the
cookie with her in the car and ate most of it, except for
the bite that I had. Sooo yummy (but also loaded with
sugar)!

At the supermarket, an employee was giving out
samples of pumpkin pie that contained whole eggs,
non-fat dry milk, and whey. Rachel tasted it and loved
it! I was beside myself, but I thought "if she wants it,
then the mind-body thing should be working." We
bought a whole pumpkin pie (containing whole eggs,
nonfat dry milk and whey) to eat for dessert that night.
We also bought some Ben and Jerry's ice cream with
egg. We would start working on that in the next few
days, but I wanted her to choose the flavor.

Amazingly, there were no issues from the cookie or
the taste of pumpkin pie. So was she allergic or was she

not? It was confusing but so exciting to watch her go through this extraordinary change.

By 4:15, Rachel ate her daily allotment of Breyers organic ice cream and felt fine. The next day, I slightly increased her carefully measured portion of ice cream to a full serving. From there on we were to start measuring a different kind of ice cream that had egg in it and eventually integrate all these foods into our normal daily life.

At this point, Rachel had gone beyond the "break even point" and was eating egg and dairy in normal portion sizes. That did not mean that our work was done – we still had to integrate the food into her diet to make it seamless – but what a huge improvement in our lifestyle!

PEDIATRICIAN ON OUR SIDE

After this incident, I contacted Rachel's pediatrician asking her to write a note to the school nurse allowing Rachel to take an Alka Seltzer Gold if she needed it while in school. I described the unconventional treatment she was undergoing and the success we were having with it.

Amazingly, Dr. Jacqui didn't chastise me for doing something that went against mainstream medicine and wrote a note to the nurse. She was thinking outside the box and cooperating with the process, something that must have been hard for her. Always so helpful, she didn't fail me now. My respect and appreciation for her was growing. I thought about our first pediatrician and shuddered, doubtful we would ever have gotten the same cooperation. He was clearly not a good match for our needs.

CHAPTER 15

The Institute for Integrative Nutrition

While my daughter was working through her food allergies, I was simultaneously doing professional work in the food allergy field. I wrote monthly newsletters and blog posts such as 'Transitioning to New Environments." My goal was to raise food allergy awareness, give guidance to parents to help them feel more confident advocating for their children, and help prevent accidental exposures to food allergies. I was also developing my own clientele.

I had been working on a presentation entitled *Food Allergy Etiquette*. Bringing my audience through the intricacies of using proper etiquette when food allergy safety was involved, it discussed situations ranging from managing food allergies at home to managing them in the homes of others. It included practical tips for communicating with restaurants, food allergy navigation during travel, and more.

In September of 2014, one of the directors of a national local parent support group sent me an email asking if I would like to speak at one of their meetings. Absolutely! I suggested my *Food Allergy Etiquette* presentation and she loved it. I presented it at a workshop in October 2014, and it was such a great success that an article was written about me in the local newspaper. To avoid ruffling any feathers, I did not mention anything about Rachel's desensitization process as I was uncertain as to how this would be received by the organization I was representing.

BACK TO SCHOOL
While talking with Alexis during one of Rachel's weekly appointments, she looked at me and asked, "What will you do once Rachel can eat anything she wants? I know you are a food allergy coach, but..."

What *will* I do? What did I want to do? I wanted to learn more about what Alexis was doing and how she did it. How could I continue working with my clients to help them avoid the things they were allergic to and keep them safe while purposefully spoon-feeding my daughter that which she was once allergic to? This was a conflict of interest and I was beginning to feel like an imposter. Also, though I was good at helping clients advocate for themselves and substitute ingredients in recipes, I needed greater understanding from a nutritional perspective of how to feed kids healthier foods.

I started looking into nutrition schools. The Institute for Integrative Nutrition (IIN), which offered a

48-week online curriculum program, looked like a good program and it would fit into my lifestyle. Most importantly, it was the school Alexis had gone to 20 or so years earlier. I enrolled.

The IIN program allowed me to better understand the allergy elimination process and what was going on with Rachel's immune system. I learned that food allergies are a multi-faceted problem that evolved over centuries. Allergies are affected by lifestyle, diet, genetics, and immune system functioning, all of which have changed more in the past century than they have during any other time period. As mentioned earlier, food allergies increased dramatically in the last 15 years. According to a study released in 2013 by the *Centers for Disease Control and Prevention*, food allergies among children increased approximately 50% between 1997 and 2011.

What was going on? Was our Western style of medicine contributing to the problem? At a Tapping World Summit Lecture, I was struck by something Dawson Church, who advanced the evolution of clinical EFT tapping, said about doctors prescribing medication. "There are two titanic forces which will collide in the next decade, HMO's which are heavily invested in wellness and the drug companies which are heavily invested in illness."

HOW MEDICINE LET RACHEL DOWN:
EAST VS. WEST

While Western medicine had let Rachel down, the therapy that Alexis was using, which integrated concepts from both Eastern and Western medicine, was working! This led me to wonder more about how the mind-body connection, positive thinking, Eastern medical techniques, and other elements that could help people.

I got some answers while attending on online lecture on December 17, 2014 about traditional and alternative medicine that was given by Frank Lipman, M.D. (www.drfranklipman.com), founder and director of the Eleven Eleven Wellness Center. He pointed out how fundamentally different Eastern and Western medical traditions treat the human body. "[There is] something in its core that views the body as a machine. In simple terms, eastern medicine views the body as a garden..."

THE UNTOLD EFFECTS OF ANTIBIOTICS

I thought back to the beginning of Rachel's allergies. When Rachel was a baby, the urologists' standard method of care to prevent kidney infections was to use prophylactic antibiotics. This was at four weeks of age, when Rachel's eczema and allergies became prevalent. At the time, nobody cautioned me that the antibiotics might affect her immune system.

Thinking back, I am sure Rachel's body knew what was happening as she was regularly vomiting the antibiotic at an early stage of this treatment. Having listened to Dr. Lipman's lecture, I became more convinced that antibiotics were at the heart of Rachel's allergies and confident that Alexis's Eastern/Western approach would boost Rachel's immune system and undo the damage done by modern Western medicine.

Something else in Dr. Lipman's lecture struck me. He explained how the body functions as one intact organism. As Rachel's specialists were each fixing only one problem in Rachel's body, her allergies may have been the resulting side effect.

How grateful I am that we found a way to resolve her allergies.

OUR SAD DIET

"People are fed by the Food Industry, which pays no attention to health, and are treated by the Health Industry which pays no attention to food."
~Wendell Berry

In large part, the food industry is to blame for the increase in food allergies. Increasingly, they have cut more and more corners, choosing profits over our well-being by making unhealthy, inexpensive "food-like" substances. This "false" food is loaded with chemicals, hormones, antibiotics, processed sugar, unhealthy fat and too much salt. All this bad stuff compromises our immune system and causes allergies and chronic and autoimmune diseases, to say nothing of causing heart disease and other serious illness, as well as reducing longevity. The Standard American Diet that most of us eat daily without questioning the consequences is SAD.

U.S. GOVERNMENT'S ROLE

Of course the food industry could not be producing the harmful food we eat daily without collusion with the U.S. Government. Here's the hard facts. The U.S. federal government subsidizes nine food industries. The number one crop that the Farm Bill subsidizes is corn. This corn gets processed into unhealthy foods like high fructose corn syrup and farmers use the surplus to feed corn to cows and other livestock.

But corn makes the animals sick. The solution? Farmers give them prophylactic antibiotics. In fact, eighty percent of the antibiotics sold in the United States are used in the meat industry. We eat the livestock, along with the unhealthy corn and the antibiotics, and this affects our immune systems by causing antibiotic resistance. When Rachel was allergic to dairy and eggs, we fed her hamburger in abundance. I now shudder at the thought and wonder how that unhealthy food was compromising her already compromised immune system. Of course, there's nothing wrong with eating meat as long as it is grass fed. But we didn't know that then.

ANTIBIOTICS AND GUT HEALTH

Introducing antibiotics into the system further compromises the developing microbiome by killing off healthy flora needed to fight disease. Let me explain further. Again, around seventy percent of our immune system is in our gut. As I've mentioned numerous times, food allergies and sensitivities are major signs that our immune systems are out of balance. An article from *Collective Evolution* explains it well: "Food, specifically undigested protein, looks just like a virus or bacteria, and our immune system creates an antibody to it. We see this in life-threatening reactions like anaphylactic shock to nuts or shellfish."

The prophylactic antibiotics my daughter was getting from four weeks old until thirteen months old were destroying her microbiome and creating an imbalance in her immune system.

THE NEWBORN GUT

Our gut contains beneficial microbes alongside thousands of different species of disease-causing microbes: bacteria, viruses, fungi and other microbes. In the healthy gut, good flora outweighs the pathogenic microbes. This balance keeps them in small colonies where they don't proliferate. In the unhealthy gut, bad flora outweighs good flora and permeates the gut wall, spreading throughout the body and brain. This appears to be what happens to virtually all children with food allergies.

Dr. Natasha Campbell–McBride, MD, a medical doctor and neurologist in the United Kingdom and author of the bestselling book, *The GAPS Diet* has studied and researched the microbiome extensively.

ANTIBIOTICS

Dr. Campbell noted the epidemic of abnormalities in the gut flora shortly after their discovery in World War II. Greatly concerned, she explained that every course of broad spectrum antibiotics wipes out the beneficial species of microbes in the gut and leaves the pathogens in there uncontrolled. Recall that Rachel first showed signs of eczema at four weeks of age, an early indication of food allergies following antibiotics given to her for hydronephrosis.

Campbell notes that while the beneficial flora recover, "... different species of it take between two weeks to two months to recover in the gut and that's a window of opportunity for various pathogens to overgrow." This is why it's so important to "reseed" your gut with fermented foods and probiotics when you're taking an antibiotic, something few doctors bother to tell you to do. Rachel's doctors certainly did not tell us this! If you aren't eating fermented foods, you should supplement with a strong probiotic on a regular basis.

BREASTFEEDING

As I mentioned earlier, breastfeeding confers protection against abnormal gut flora. Breastfed babies develop entirely different gut flora compared to bottle-fed babies.

How fortunate that I breastfed Rachel until she was 15 months old. Of note, Dr. Campbell discovered that as babies received many courses of antibiotics throughout their childhood, the abnormalities in their gut flora further deepened. Such abnormalities were further exacerbated by these woman having taken birth control pills which, explains Dr. Campbell, have a devastating effect on the gut flora.

In addition to bottle feeding, Dr. Campbell discovered that antibiotic overuse, the use of the contraceptive pill, processed junk food, and excessive consumption of high fructose corn syrup further set the stage for increasingly abnormal gut flora with each passing generation. Little wonder that food allergies have been on the rise.

PASSING ON BAD GUT FLORA

Mothers pass on their microbiome as the newborn passes through the birth canal, Campbell explains.

"...the baby acquires its gut flora at the time of birth, when the baby goes through the birth canal of the mother.

So what lives in mom's vagina? It's a very richly populated area of a woman's body. The vaginal flora comes from the bowel. So if the mother has abnormal gut flora, she will have abnormal flora in her birth canal. Fathers are not exempt because fathers also have gut flora, and that gut flora populates their groin and they share their groin flora with the mother on a regular basis."

Unfortunately, I was one of these. I was not breast-fed, took long-term antibiotics as a child for my hydronephrosis, and was on birth control pills for many years. As you may recall, I suffered frequently from yeast infections. So not only were antibiotics killing the good flora in Rachel's gut, but she was likely born with poor gut flora because I had insufficient gut flora in my gut.

Again, it is very, very fortunate that I had a normal vaginal delivery and breastfed Rachel for as long as I did. Notes Campbell,

> *While the baby is breastfed, despite the fact that the baby has acquired abnormal gut flora from the mom, there will be some protection. But as soon as the breastfeeding stops that protection stops as well.*"

As you recall, that was exactly what happened. As soon as I starting weaning, Rachel's allergies got worse.

Further, the establishment of normal gut flora in the first 20 days or so of life plays a *crucial role* in appropriate maturation of the baby's immune system. Babies who are born with abnormal gut flora are left with compromised immune systems.

WORK TRANSITION

All this information was adding up and in March 2015 I started working with clients as an Integrative Nutrition Health Coach. My first client's goal was to be able to give her son healthy snacks when he got home from school. She wanted healthy snack foods to sustain him until dinner, and she wanted to learn more about which options were most nutritious. Enthusiastic about the nutritional and lifestyle options I was able to offer, she excitedly implemented my suggestions. I gained another client who wanted to lower her cholesterol, and I started working with another who wanted to find foods that would be easier for him to digest.

*"Every time you eat or drink, you are either feeding disease
or fighting it."*
~Heather Morgan, MS, NLC.

In April, another health coach practitioner that I
met in NYC at an IIN conference introduced me to the
Allergies and Your Gut website that proved to be very informative in helping me to understand how our diet
makes a huge difference in our health.

This website gave me more information on how
probiotics help us balance our gut. I also learned that,
while most people think you get probiotics from supplements, we are better off getting them from fermented
foods, like raw sauerkraut, kefir and kombucha as they
contain far more of the good gut flora our body needs.
Natasha Campbell's GAPS diet focuses on eating loads
of fermented foods daily. The website also discussed
how sugar, white breads and processed foods are like
crack for our bodies; they are addictive and slowly destroy our immune system.

FEEDING RACHEL JUNK
Just as I felt like an imposter telling my clients what
foods to avoid while Rachel was increasing her tolerance
to those foods, I also felt like an imposter for encouraging healthy eating while I was feeding my daughter way
too much sugar and white flour. Unfortunately, sugary
sweets were the easiest way to expand Rachel's exposure; it was easier to get her to eat baked goods with
eggs than pancakes or French toast. For this reason, we
gave Rachel increasingly larger portions of cakes, cook-

ies and brownies. And though I would not recommend this to my health coaching clients, I was pleased that Rachel was able to eat these foods at all.

CHAPTER 16

Social Eating:
Food Diary, Part 3

1-31-15

At a Bar Mitzvah luncheon, Rachel had the choice of French toast sticks or macaroni and cheese at the kids' food table. She chose the latter, and I put a large spoonful of mac and cheese on her plate. This was risky as she had never eaten it before and we had no idea if she could eat it safely. Also I had not read any labels, so I didn't know how many chemicals it contained.

Praying she would be OK, I told her to eat a few noodles slowly. I noticed dark circles under her eyes and became momentarily concerned but quickly realized that they were from the previous night's sleepover party with her girlfriends! I kept asking, "Are you OK?" And she kept replying, "I'm fine, Mom!" behaving like your typical eleven-year-old kid.

Next, she proceeded to the dessert table; she had brownies and a small taste of key lime pie. Letting the healthy things go for this occasion, I did manage to get some watermelon in her.

We had reached a new plateau! A year ago, or even a few months earlier, we would have had to bring food with us to the Bar Mitzvah or call the caterer to find out what was on the menu. On this day, we just showed up and our daughter tried something new for the first time! Imagine an eleven-year-old girl eating macaroni and cheese for the first time in her life. Such a happy occasion!

On the way home, we said the *shehekianu* prayer. This is a prayer that you say when something new and exciting happens in your life or for the first time in the year as a way of showing gratitude. Generally it is said for special occasions like an anniversary or a birthday. This day was very much a special occasion, so we had a small family spiritual experience in the car on the way home.

2-1-15

The next day, after eating macaroni and cheese for the first time in her life, Rachel ate a homemade kind of mac and cheese at a super bowl party. This was a completely different mac and cheese than the day before. Rachel just shoveled a helping onto her plate. I thought that amount was plenty, but then she shoveled some more onto her plate and said I was being overprotective.

She was absolutely fine!

This day's dairy intake was unbelievable:

Breakfast – 4 pieces or a full serving of European milk chocolate

AM snack – A specifically measured portion of Amy's frozen pizza for the first time ever!

PM snack – Her allotted portion of Ben & Jerry's Mint Chocolate Cookie ice cream.

Dinner – macaroni and cheese at a super bowl party, a brownie with cream cheese, half of a chocolate cupcake, and a butter cookie.

Though it was hard to give her so many foods spaced two hours apart, we were home more than usual that week because we had two days with no school due to a snowstorm. It all worked out fine.

This day constituted about five months into the desensitization process for dairy and about thirteen months into the allergy elimination process.

2-5-15

Rachel started eating whipped cream on her ice cream. Later in the week she would start eating Abbott's frozen custard, starting with half of a kiddie size and eventually progressing to a full kiddie size. And she started bringing Horizon organic mozzarella cheese sticks to school for lunch!

We learned that Rachel's friend was having pizza at his birthday party the next day.

In the past, birthday parties needed preparation. I sometimes bought Rachel sushi or dairy-free pizza covered in foil with her name saying "RACHEL's DO NOT TOUCH!" But times were changing and she would now have pizza at her friend's birthday party.

To be safe without me there, we did a trial at home. I called the friend's mom to find out what pizza store the birthday party would order from and Rachel ate it with no problems! Amazing. We put a video on Facebook for our friends and family to see her eating her first bite of commercial pizza! I did however insist that she eat something healthy first before eating the pizza and she ate four baby spinach leaves. We didn't put *that* on Facebook!

The next day, she ate a slice of pizza at the birthday party, shocking and amazing her friends. One of them asked "What's going to happen to you?" Nothing happened.

As for me, I could no longer contain my excitement about her progress and shared my news about our allergy elimination process in my February Newsletter "There is Hope!" You could say that I came out of the closet.

2-16-15
For breakfast, Rachel tried peaches and cottage cheese. She didn't like the cottage cheese – "too lumpy." For a snack, she had Ben & Jerry's Karamel Sutra Core ice cream.

I was constantly trying to balance my values as a health coach with my concerns as a mother and our perseverance with the desensitization process. Many of the new foods she was eating contained sugar. Rachel was much more likely to eat ice cream than a non-sugary dairy product, or a butter cookie than egg fried rice.

We had a conversation about Ben and Jerry's being a non-GMO product. I explained how non-GMO products are much healthier than GMO products because of the chemicals and the way they are processed. Rachel piped in, "So GMO products are so unhealthy, but this fatty ice cream with whipped cream is very healthy!" My daughter doesn't miss a beat. How do you explain to a 12 year old why I preferred that she had healthy fat than sugar? Oh, well. I learned to pick my battles and let her eat what she wanted. She needed to consume the foods to which she had created a tolerance so we could continue to build her tolerance to more foods. We would work on the healthy piece later.

3-13-15
Another great milestone. My sixth grader bought lunch at school for the first time in several years! It had been so long since she bought lunch at school that it took me a day to find her cafeteria code back in her kindergarten file. I had transferred most of her lunch money to her sister's account as, in the past, buying lunch at school was too risky and I never thought she would; we couldn't trust the issues of cross contact.

In kindergarten, she ate a bagel with sunflower butter to learn how to navigate the cafeteria system. On this day she ate the main course; a cheese quesadilla.

One friend slapped the palm of his hand on his forehead in disbelief. Another concerned friend asked, "What's going to happen to you?" A third friend exclaimed "I didn't know you buy lunch!"

Granted, the lunches that were sold and prepared at school were less healthy and less nutritious than the lunches that I put so much love into at home. But how freeing! After all, it's very important for pre-teens to fit in with their peers. Now she would.

3-27-15
Today the cafeteria was serving mac-n-cheese. I was a bit nervous as I knew it was not organic and of course asked her how it was and if anything happened. Vaguely, she responded, "Good," like a typical tween. Apparently nothing happened.

3-30-15
That evening our family went to a burrito place for dinner. Our daughter would normally just order a beef burrito without cheese and we normally would have had a conversation with the staff about her allergies. On this night, she asked me "Can I have cheese on my burrito?"

"You can have anything you like, sweetie."

"Anything you like" went a little too far because she also drank an unhealthy sugary orange soda from the fountain. I let it go. Hard to do but necessary as I knew how important it was to promote her budding autonomy.

PASSOVER 2015

Eggs are symbolic for new signs of life each year as the birth of spring brings on both the Easter and Passover holidays. But in our house eggs had never been abundant because of the fear of a visit to the emergency room. Through the years, I learned to improvise to make our Seder "safe" for our egg-allergic daughter. I would make a squash soufflé, a family recipe in which I substituted all six eggs for other rising-type ingredients. Fortunately, the kids always loved this recipe and Rachel often begged for more; I confess it was made with a cup of sugar.

This year though we would celebrate Passover eating eggs as a family. It was our first, and I was excited! To insure we would not have any surprise processing episodes I made my famous squash soufflé recipe the week before Passover with non-Passover (regular) flour.

One day before the kids got home from school, I mixed up the ingredients for the soufflé, including all six eggs. As it baked, the whole house smell like a freshly baked cake; soooo good! After I removed the lasagna-sized pan from the oven and let it cool, I cut the soufflé into 20 bite-sized pieces. A quick calculation proved .3 of an egg in each piece. It was hard to get Rachel to eat eggs even though she was no longer allergic to them, but this would be a good way for her to get exposure. Yet, in spite of loving this recipe in the past, she took two bites and said, "It tastes like egg. I'm good."

Uuuugh! What was I going to do with a not-kosher-for-Passover lasagna-sized tin of soufflé? My younger daughter ate two pieces, and I ate two pieces. My husband, who's not a sugar fan, wasn't interested.

The next morning, I warmed up a piece and Rachel ate it while watching television. Great. Maybe my family will actually finish it. But no. After saying it was good, Rachel would eat no more. Being the mother of a child going through allergy elimination is an ongoing challenge. How do you get your child to eat foods she must eat but which to her are distasteful?

Now, I had to decide how to bake my soufflé for the Seder so it was less eggy. Should I put all six eggs or substitute some of the eggs? I decided to put four organic eggs into the soufflé and substitute the last two with 2 tablespoons of flaxseed and 1/3 cup of warm water. This would calculate to .2 or less than a quarter of an egg per slice.

After all my painstaking labor, Rachel never even tasted it at the Seder, as she felt too full after eating my homemade organic chicken soup. She did though eat two large egg-containing matzo balls in her chicken soup, so she did have some egg. As she was never able to eat matzo balls before on Passover, this alone was a

FROM ANAPHYLAXIS TO BUTTERCREAM

milestone. And there was no processing. Sigh of relief. We were safe.

But, just when I thought her allergy reactions were over there was another episode. The second night of Passover, we made plans to join our synagogue for their annual congregational Seder. After the Rabbi started the community Seder, they started serving soup with matzo balls that had fully cooked egg. Rachel gobbled up two helpings of matzo balls. That was one matzo ball for lunch and two for dinner; three for the day. We were doing well.

We finished our dinner, sang a few songs, and it was time for dessert. The dessert was chocolate mousse. I went to another table to say hello to some friends. As I began chatting, my younger daughter came over to me and announced, "Rachel is not feeling well."

Oh no! I calmly rushed over to the table in a diplomatic manner so as not to alarm the friends with whom I was chatting. Rachel had just eaten the chocolate mousse and her tongue itched, her stomach hurt and she felt a little itchy. Fortunately, her eyes weren't swollen and her nose was not running.

She already had two Alka Seltzer Gold tablets that day, so I wasn't sure if it was the two matzo balls that she had eaten an hour before or the immediate response to the chocolate mousse. But if the mousse set it off, this was a precedent as it happened a few minutes after ingestion and typically processing occurred about an hour after ingestion.

Perhaps it was the last straw on the camel's back. In addition to the matzo balls and the chocolate mousse, she had also eaten frozen yogurt earlier in the day and perhaps all three were too much for her immune system. Further, in addition to having a lot of egg, the mousse contained an egg/dairy combination. And there were other possible factors. It was close to her bedtime and this made her more vulnerable to processing.

Whatever the reasons, I didn't want to take any chances. So I grabbed one chewable antihistamine from my pocketbook and gave it to her. She chewed it and swallowed it with some water and we did her mantra and EFT (Emotional Freedom Technique) tapping to manage the negative emotions associated with the processing episode. She said she felt a little better.

Nevertheless, I was intent on solving the mystery. My husband put the remainder of the chocolate mousse from her plate into a container to bring with us to Alexis's office on our next visit, and Rachel and I went into the kitchen to find out the ingredients from the caterer. Unfortunately, he bought it from a bakery and didn't have the exact ingredients but he was certain it contained chocolate, heavy cream, eggs, and sugar. By the time we got home, Rachel was fine and went to bed.

Though this incident was frightening, it was helpful in that we found some things she was processing with egg and willing to eat. I now had to find out either where to buy this mousse from a bakery or make it myself so we could continue working on it.

4-9-15
Our next appointment with Alexis helped to clear up some of the mystery. She said the chocolate mousse from Saturday night probably had undercooked egg, along with Rachel having eaten the mousse on the same day that she processed frozen yogurt.

Rachel now seemed past the processing. On the way to see Alexis, she ate two cheese sticks in the car. Once we arrived, she ate the remainder of the frozen yogurt -- a few tablespoons. After she ate it Alexis had Rachel do her mantra and tapping. Nothing happened and Alexis considered this positive imprinting.

So what was it? The frozen custard? It seemed unlikely. The next day Rachel ate half a mini black raspberry custard pie for dessert without any processing. Was it the mousse or the yogurt? It was hard to know. Even though one of the differences between the frozen yogurt and the custard was whey, there were also a lot of chemicals in the products and the chemicals used to process the ingredients in frozen yogurt and custard were different.

"FALSE" FOOD
All these chemicals in our food upset me. Why should her body have to get used to chemicals? Should

I not just be feeding her whole, unprocessed, unrefined healthy food?

This was an ongoing dilemma for me. I was learning so much about how bad the food most of us eat in the standard American diet. Yet, I felt compelled to continue to give her "junk." As I previously reiterated, she was a preteen and wanting to be like the other kids, including eating what her friends ate. After she had been deprived of doing so her whole life, I felt it important that she be enabled.

Further, while at home I could make the food as healthy as possible, I couldn't control what Rachel ate outside the house. If she didn't eat this highly processed food so her body could learn to process it, she could conceivably eat something when away from home that could cause a reaction. Also, Alexis had set up a specific regimen for us and I didn't want to deviate from it. For these reasons, I felt it was far more important at this point to rid her of her allergies and focus on eating healthy down the road.

RACHEL'S ANNUAL PHYSICAL: APRIL 14, 2015

On April 14th we spent half an hour with the pediatrician, Dr. Jacqui, to discuss Rachel's yearlong progress. After thanking her for the note she wrote to the school nurse and expressing how much we appreciated her help, I read to her the amazing list of Rachel's milestones and accomplishments.

- **5-1-14** - Started straight egg.
- **6-5-14** - Started baked-in egg.
- **Month of July 2014** - half of a hard-boiled egg and one baked-in product containing egg every day at overnight camp.
- **7-30-14** - Ate French toast.
- **9-5-14** - Started introducing dairy (yogurt).
- **11-18-14** - Switched from yogurt to ice cream slowly.
- **12-5-14** - Brought Back to Nature crispy cheddar crackers to school for lunch.
- **2-5-15** - Ordered pizza for dinner.
- **2-6-15** - Ate pizza at birthday party.
- **3-13-15** - Bought lunch at school.

I also shared our "setbacks" with the doctor.

- **6-17-14** - First time we processed from a baked-in cupcake.
- **12-11-14** - Rachel did not go to school because of major processing.

Dr. Jacqui asked numerous questions to understand the process. I answered them as best I could.

As usual, Dr. Jacqui was positive and supportive. Her response was simply, "If it works...!" I was so thankful to have found someone from the medical community who was open to other ways of healing. I told Dr. Jacqui that we would not go back to the allergist because of the letter she wrote, expressing disapproval of the process.

Dr. Jacqui asked me what she should put on Rachel's medical forms. This astounded me. Based on my conversation with another mom whose child graduated from this program, the doctor had not been able to take the allergies off of the health forms because she either hadn't been re-tested or hadn't tested negative. Our doctor actually asked me how it should be handled. I wasn't expecting that.

I wasn't sure we should take the allergies off of her health form entirely since she was still having some processing with products such as raw egg but at least we knew it was an option.

Dr. Jacqui told us it wasn't a good idea to eat raw egg anyway because of the risk of salmonella. Then she wrote up Rachel's new allergy action plan:

"Allergens: egg, milk, and mustard. She may eat moderate amounts of these foods and take Alka Seltzer Gold if symptomatic. She still has EpiPen/Benadryl available."

This was right on! I gave a copy of the new health memorandum to the school nurse. When my daughter came home from school, she told me that egg was no longer on her allergy list in the school cafeteria. We were making great strides.

Success happens in little steps along the way, yet hardly ever in a straight line.
This was the phrase that kept me going throughout the process. Nothing is ever perfect, but we do succeed.

I remember seeing it on a coffee mug about 25 years ago while working at my first job. It has become my mantra ever since. It was time for Rachel and me to take a deep breath and appreciate all the progress we successfully achieved.

4-20-15
We were visiting my in-laws in Pittsburgh. For lunch, Rachel ate Kraft macaroni and cheese that we made in my mother-in-law's kitchen. I don't believe Rachel had ever eaten this before. After fervently eating several bites, her facial expression changed and she abruptly stopped. I knew something was wrong. She took a few more small bites and then stopped again. A red flag for sure. As we were all eating together, I didn't say anything so as to not cause any drama.

She went into the other room, and after I cleaned up some of the dishes, I went to check on her. I found her lying on the bed reading a book. Her eyes were swollen, and she was blowing her nose. I was concerned. If she knew something was wrong, why did she ignore her symptoms and fail to take action? Why didn't she come get me to tell me something was wrong? Clearly, she waited for me to initiate any resolution. I still had to be right on her.

I put two Alka Seltzer Gold tablets in some water and gave her the glass to drink. She put the glass down without drinking it and went into the bathroom to get a tissue. This was frustrating as the sooner she got the medicine into her system, the sooner the symptoms would go away. But, again, to avoid any drama, I let it go.

She drank the Alka Seltzer Gold when she came back and we did her mantra and tapping. At that point she had three small hives on her stomach, and none on her back or arms, but she started itching. Half an hour later, her hives were a little worse, so I gave her one chewable antihistamine. She could have had more Alka Seltzer Gold or two antihistamine, but I thought that was enough.

An hour after the antihistamine, the hives looked a lot better. They weren't red and swollen, but the bumps were still visible.

Again, I suspected the problem was all the chemicals in the processed macaroni and cheese and we needed to work on this. These same reactions were happening with frozen yogurt and custard, again all highly processed. The reactions did not happen with pizza, which was freshly made and minimally processed.

As usual, I felt horrifically conflicted. Knowing how unhealthy highly processed food was even for a perfectly healthy body, I wanted to tell her to eat only organic ingredients. What was all this junk doing to my daughter? Could it be doing a disservice to her in the long run?

But I was loathe to stop her from eating what she wished. I kept telling myself that her body had to learn to process this food because she would be eating it at camp and school. So, reluctantly I gave in as I knew I couldn't always be in charge of her food.

4-27-15
    I didn't have time to make Rachel's lunch, so she bought lunch at school. I had no idea what was on the menu this day. Then, while making tortellini for her sister for dinner, I found out that she had cheese tortellini with meatballs, garlic sauce and parmesan cheese for lunch and didn't want it again. "I don't like tortellini. Besides, I had it for lunch," she said.

    Phew! What a great allergy accomplishment! She ate tortellini at school for lunch and nothing happened. We had come so far. Not only didn't I know what she ate that day, I had no idea what she ate or how much she ate all week. On Friday, I was surprised to learn that she ate the fish sticks, but like the kids say "don't question it" so I didn't. I also found an empty Dorito chip bag left in my car when I picked her up from play practice at the end of the day that she undoubtedly got from the school cafeteria.

    All was fine with me. She was showing age-appropriate independence that grew daily, and with it increasing confidence.

    I also reminded myself that I had to choose my battles, and stopping her from eating junk food could wait. What was important was that, in spite of all the processed food, it was a seamless week.

5-1-15

Today represented another milestone. We had eggs and dairy mostly under our belt and started working on mustard using Annie's Honey Mustard Dressing – a home-grown and organic salad dressing.

I served her a plate of carrots, crackers and mustard-filled measuring spoons that she ate by way of dipping. I was thrilled that she was consuming a veggie as part of her therapy. By the third day Rachel commented on the number of baby carrots she had to eat to consume the amount of mustard required for the day, but she ate it. As I had with the other allergens, I would check off each day in my notebook as she accomplished her mustard goal.

We were almost done with dairy, but were still working on the chemical-laden and highly processed mac-n-cheese and ice cream. On Saturday just before lunch I gave her a stick of organic mozzarella cheese. Around 3:00 I asked her if she wanted some mac-n-cheese. She said no because she didn't like the highly processed kind, so instead I made her some of the Annie's creamy deluxe organic mac-n-cheese, where you boil the shells and then add the cheese sauce from the foil bag.

After preparing it, I left the cooked product on the counter in a glass container and told her to take as much as she would like. I didn't watch her take it or eat it, but when I went downstairs she said she had eaten about half a bowl. She said it tasted more like the highly processed kind and that she didn't like it as much as the frozen Amy's organic kind that she had the other night. She also said she wasn't hungry, which made sense because she had been snacking all day.

Nothing happened.

During this week, my daughter, my mother and I went out for dinner and Rachel ordered the meatloaf stuffed with fresh mozzarella cheese, served with mashed potatoes. I got emotional seeing her eat cheese. She ate the bread with olive oil that had parmesan cheese mixed in as well, even more dairy! We've come a long way.

"It's such a pleasure to go out to eat with her. I can't believe the difference in her now that she can eat everything!" my mother beamed.

5-4-15
Seasonal allergies were kicking in and Rachel's eyes were itchy in the morning so I gave her an Allertec, an antihistamine (a generic version of Zyrtec cetirizine hydrochloride – 10 mg).

I bought some organic mango kefir that has 22 grams of sugar per 8 ounce serving. After eating her carrots and honey mustard dressing, she drank about 4 ounces of the kefir. I wished she liked dairy without added sugar, but she now preferred the kefir over yogurt for breakfast. That was fine with me as kefir is a fermented drink. As previously mentioned, the more probiotics daily the stronger her microbiome and, ultimately her immune system.

The next day, it occurred to me that I no longer had to get up before 6:30 a.m. to measure my daughter's allotted portion for the day or make her lunch. She was eating a protein bar for breakfast that contained whey and other ingredients. This could certainly be improved, but for now it was working. She was buying lunch at school every day, including the pizza sticks. This meant less weight in her backpack, but also letting go of part of my mothering.

How did I feel about this? Well of course wonderful but also gripped with the reality of my baby growing up and not needing her mother as much. And this, as any mother knows, brings with it feelings of pathos.

ENCOURAGING RACHEL TO TAKE CONTROL OF HER ALLERGIES

On May 8, 2015 around 8:15 p.m., I noticed some symptoms, but I wasn't sure if they were "processing" from the custard or environmental allergies from the tree pollen. Everyone was itchy and sneezy that day. Even I was blinking my eyes a little. My ears felt clogged and kept popping and I usually never have any allergy symptoms. I didn't say anything.

She did not have a Zyrtec that morning, and I noticed that she was coughing, blowing her nose, rubbing her eyes and one of her eyes was beginning to get red from rubbing.

Was she just tired? "Are you OK?" I asked her.

She said she needed her inhaler. We were upstairs near the bathroom, where the inhaler was kept. I said, "Let's go downstairs and talk about this before you take a shower."

We went downstairs to the kitchen where we kept the medicine. I wanted her to decide what to do about her coughing and runny nose. She needed to learn to take control of her own body; how else could we trust her to eat without supervision?

"I didn't have a Zyrtec this morning," she said. "Can I have one?"

"Yes, but do you think you need an Alka?"

"NO!" she shouted. "Just give me a Zyrtec." How do you train a 12-year-old kid who should know her body from an allergy standpoint to determine what she needed? Luckily my husband piped in... "A Zyrtec is not going to help you immediately. It's not very strong, but it will last for longer."

"It's not that bad," she said, in apparent denial that the symptoms might be from the ice cream she had eaten well over an hour ago.

She was right. It wasn't bad. It was just flushing well over an hour after eating a regular size black raspberry custard in a cone. Her body was getting used to it, or it could have been exacerbated by the tree pollen. But whatever it was I didn't want her to take any chances and I didn't want it to get worse. I gave her the Zyrtec with some water.

"Do you think you should still have an Alka?" I asked.

My husband intervened to help settle the mother-daughter battle. "If you took your long-acting inhaler a few days ago and then you didn't take it for a few days that could make your allergies worse. You need to be consistent to prevent symptoms or take the red one. The Alka is not going to hurt you if you take it, but if you don't take it your symptoms could get worse."

We waited, every second feeling like an hour as I couldn't force her to take the Alka Seltzer Gold.

Finally, she said "OK."

I plopped two tablets into a few ounces of water and like usual, it sat there on the table and she stared at it. I sat there next to her and didn't say a word. I just closed my eyes and remained calm. Another minute went by. I was just going to wait. *She needs to do this. I cannot force it down her.*

I broke and asked her if she was going to drink it. "YES!" But she didn't drink it. She was rubbing her eyes. I waited some more.

And then she took a sip, rubbed her eyes some more. It took forever for her to drink it down one sip at a time but she finally did and then did her mantra and tapping.

No more symptoms. Just one red eye and blowing her nose. It was almost 9:00 p.m.. Time to get ready for bed. She did her inhaler, brushed her teeth, put on her pajamas and got into bed. She was tired. Whatever was happening wasn't bad. It just was.

The next day her eyes were a little puffy for most of the day. Maybe the whole ordeal was just because of environmental allergies. The same thing happened last year at camp. She had reactions then and we didn't know why, but that was at the end of June and this was the beginning of May.

The very next night, Saturday, May 9, 2015, Rachel had eight sixth-graders over for an overnight birthday party. We started the night by ordering a pizza from one of our favorite local places. It was a beautiful night, and we ate outside in the backyard by the fire pit.

After the pizza, we sugared the kids up on s'mores marshmallows, milk chocolate, and graham crackers. Everyone had a blast! A little after 8 p.m. the kids watched *Now You See Me* starring Mark Ruffalo and Morgan Freeman, and I gave everyone popcorn.

A little after 9 p.m. we asked everyone if they would like to take a break from the movie to have ice cream cake. The response was unanimous. I had taken the frozen custard cake out of the freezer and left it in the fridge a little over an hour before, so I was hoping it would be defrosted just enough to slice. Trying to avoid any repeat issues from the night before and knowing that it had been 24 hours since the last Zyrtec, I asked my daughter if she would take one. She said "OK." It wasn't going to do much in the next few minutes, but at least if it was just environmental we would get ahead of it.

We sang *Happy Birthday*, and I cut the frozen custard cake. It had been a long while since I had ever cut an ice cream cake for someone in our family. The cake said "Happy Birthday Rachel" on three separate lines, so I cut off the "Rachel" part which would leave about ⅔ of the cake for the 8 kids and two adults (including me). Salivating for the salted caramel and chocolate ice cream cake, I purposely cut the pieces small as everyone had already had enough sugar including the s'mores two hours ago, and it was 9 p.m., a little late for Rachel to have ice cream.

After singing "Happy Birthday" and finishing the movie, the kids went upstairs on the third floor for their sleepover portion of the party.

At 11 p.m. I woke up because I heard someone coughing. Even though there were seven kids sleeping in the finished attic, I was sure it was our daughter. At 4:20 AM I heard her coughing again.

The next morning, I asked if she was okay --"I heard you coughing last night."

"I was not coughing!"

Uuuugh! "Yes you were!"

"OK, maybe in my sleep." I wasn't going to fight this one.

Her eyes were swollen, but her nose wasn't running. Perhaps she was just tired. Maybe the day before was mostly seasonal and a little bit of processing; as we say "her cup runneth over" and her immune system had been slightly overloaded.

In the end, her birthday party went well! Her allergies were not hindering her lifestyle. But I needed to take a chill pill and stop overanalyzing her symptoms to try to figure out what was causing them. Rachel was learning to take control of her own body; I needed to work on letting go.

CHAPTER 17

Preparing for Summer 2015

FILLING OUT CAMP FORMS

Every year I had to fill out a new batch of paperwork before sending both of my daughters to camp. With a huge liability issue at stake, the camp had to be thorough. Of course, I also had high stakes. I had to figure out how to let the camp know that Rachel could now eat the things she was once allergic to without causing concern but, at the same time, watch her because her body was still adjusting to them.

Filling in the forms hit home on how enormously our lives had changed. Herewith is what I wrote in the forms.

<u>Medical Forms:</u>
Food allergies: **eggs, dairy, mustard**

Please describe the reaction and how it is treated:
Rachel can eat large amounts of the things she was once al-

lergic to (eggs/dairy) because she has recently gone through a systematic desensitization therapy process with success! She is fine with organic ingredients, however she is still "processing" things like Kraft cheese and undercooked egg (chocolate mousse) in large amounts. The "processing" reactions can happen immediately or 1-2 hours after she has eaten it and can be exacerbated by environmental allergies. She will present with swollen eyes or a bump on the lip, then these symptoms can escalate to itchiness and hives. Rachel should get 2 Alka Seltzer Gold dissolved in water. She should also do her mantra and tapping. If hives are already present when being treated, she can also have up to 2 chewable Benadryl tablets. She should then rest for about an hour. The Benadryl will make her sleepy.

Is there a risk of anaphylactic reaction?: *Yes - this is still possible.*

Environmental allergies: *trees mold and grass.*

Please describe the reaction and how it is treated: *Itchy eyes, blowing nose, coughing. She can use her long acting and short acting inhaler as appropriate and take Zyrtec™ every day.*

Parent Forms:
I filled out a required questionnaire from parent to director. This was the same camp, for the third year in a row, but each year the forms and questions were revised and slightly different.

Q: Are there any health or behavioral issues of which we should be aware? If yes, please describe in detail.

A: *Rachel is now eating all baked products including cake, crackers, cookies, and brownies. She can eat yogurt, buttercream, pizza, ice cream, mozzarella cheese, and milk chocolate. Regarding straight eggs: She ate ½ a hardboiled egg every morning at camp last summer, but now she says she hates the taste of eggs, so I struggle to get her to eat them. The more she eats these foods, the greater her tolerance. Instead of avoiding these foods, we are encouraging her to eat them. It's a whole new mind set.*

As a suggestion, Rachel should eat half a serving when trying something new to get her body used to it.

5-14-15
By this time, I felt I could relax. Rachel was a normal child, or should I say tween, who could eat a normal diet. And then, out of the blue, her second major processing incident happened – the only other time during the entire desensitization process that I contemplated giving her epinephrine.

On the way home from my friend's office, Rachel and I had a nice conversation about spirituality. I was astounded because this was a 12-year-old kid who spent most of her free time lying on the floor in the family room watching *My Little Pony* on her iPad.

She had just eaten half a protein bar (10 grams of protein). The protein bar contained: *Protein blend (Whey*

protein isolate, milk protein isolate), isothermal-Oligosaccha-
rides which are prebiotic fibers derived from plant sources,
Erythritol, water, unsweetened chocolate, almonds, cocoa, co-
coa butter, sea salt, steviol glycosides (stevia), natural flavors.

Suddenly she said she was itchy; her nose was
stuffed and she said she needed her inhaler. What was
going on!? I was worried, as I was still driving and we
wouldn't be home for another eight minutes. To clear
whatever emotional blockage she was having, I suggested that she do her mantra and tapping. She screamed
"NO!" and got hysterical!

I had no idea where this was coming from since we
were just having such a nice conversation about spiritual practice. I pulled the Alka Seltzer Gold out of my
pocketbook but I had no way to give it to her while I was
driving. We had water, but no cup. I called my husband
from the car and asked him to get two "Alkas" ready
for her to drink when we got home. I was calm, but he
knew this was serious.

In hindsight, I should have told Rachel to take a
Benadryl from her epi belt which was accessible to her
from her backpack in the car. She wasn't thinking either. If I was with her, she expected me to take care
of her. "What will happen when she goes to camp," I
worried.

When we got home, she drank the "Alka" Ed had
ready for her. But we didn't catch the reaction in time.

She now had a few hives and then a full blown out rash all over her entire body.

At this point, nothing that she had eaten should have caused a problem but it did. Why? It appeared to be the whey protein. To begin, she could now eat two organic mozzarella sticks without any problem and each mozzarella stick contained 8 grams of protein making that 16 grams of protein in total. Half of the protein bar, which she ate and processed had only 10 grams of protein but it was whey blend isolate, a processed protein and that apparently tripped her immune system. This is a bad and potentially harmful protein for all bodies as it is overly acidifying and lacking alkalizing minerals, naturally occurring vitamins, and lipids, which are lost in the processing.

Further, as Dr. Mercola explains:

"Many cheap whey protein isolates are produced from acid cheese ....which is a cheap way to separate whey from the curd. Most of these whey products are rated below pet foods because of the inferior quality of the protein, which is actually more of a nitrogen waste product than one that will produce health benefits that are mentioned in the featured study."

To add further insult to her immune system, she was processing environmental allergies at the same time, especially with birch tree pollen. Further, she had had booster vaccines for Menactra and Tdap, over a month prior and these immunizations were still taxing her immune system. Altogether, they took her over the edge.

This processing incident gave me a sleepless night. But it didn't seem to bother Rachel. Like clockwork, the next morning, Rachel rode her bike to school with her friends as if nothing ever happened. That's my Rachel!

5-19-15
As far as I knew, Rachel hadn't eaten a whole egg in a long time. On this day, she said she was looking forward to it as she was having it for lunch at school. My husband said "If she is looking forward to eating egg, then I'm not complaining." She did eat it all the time, but not as straight egg and mostly in ice cream. When she came home from school, I asked her what she had for lunch. She said "the egg and cheese sandwich, but I'm pretty sure that it was imitation egg because I liked it. It didn't taste like egg."

I looked up the ingredients via the school's lunch program: (egg patty, cheese and slice of turkey Canadian bacon or pork sausage patty) on English muffin or bagel. Egg patty contains modified food starch (a processed food). It was egg! She would eat egg at school with her friends, but not at home – another example of mind-body connection. To be like her friends, she ignored her palate. At home, she was free to be totally herself.

One part of me was thrilled that she was buying lunch at school, even though I had no idea what she was eating. Yet another part was apprehensive. She had just had another major processing episode from protein isolate. Perhaps food served at school contained this ingredient. Should I be so complacent? I felt confused.

To be safe, I always had my cell phone with me and tried to not be more than 20 minutes away from being able to pick her up should the necessity arise. Let's say I felt a cautious optimism.

MEMORIAL DAY WEEKEND
Friday night our family walked into town after dinner to get frozen custard. Rachel ate one of the mini pies with black raspberry frozen custard and a graham cracker crust.

Nothing happened.

On Saturday I was at the hair salon and texted her: "You need to eat something before going to your friend's house. What will you eat?" Her response: "idk,"
At the friend's house, she ate leftover taco meat and cheddar cheese on a hamburger bun.

Nothing happened.

At home for dinner, she ate Belle & Evans organic chicken marinated in mustard. She was fine. Then I bought 4" waffle cups at Whole Foods lined with chocolate. She ate this filled with cookies and cream frozen custard and topped with whipped cream. "Delicious!" she uttered.

Nothing happened.

On Sunday, we had a BBQ party with 18 people at our house. She had a cheeseburger with cheddar cheese (Adams Reserve, New York extra sharp cheddar: pasteurized milk, cheese culture, salt, enzymes, annatto (vegetable color) aged over 12 months.) No chemicals.

She also had a small slice of ice cream cake that we had ordered to celebrate three of our friends' birthdays. The first time she had eaten this same ice cream cake, she had a bump on her lip just from tasting the cake batter ice cream. We had come so far! Then, after eating the slice of cake she had a few s'mores with milk chocolate. Lots of sugar.

Nothing happened.

On Monday afternoon at my friend Jessica's BBQ, Rachel ate two ice cream sandwiches. Jessica, who had a son with multiple food allergies shrieked, "Oh my God. I can't believe my eyes. She's eating an ice cream sandwich!"

"I know!" I said. "I still can't believe it either. Every time I see it, I still get emotional with that bittersweet momentary sense of panic. I'm so grateful everything is now OK!"

PART FOUR
GRADUATION

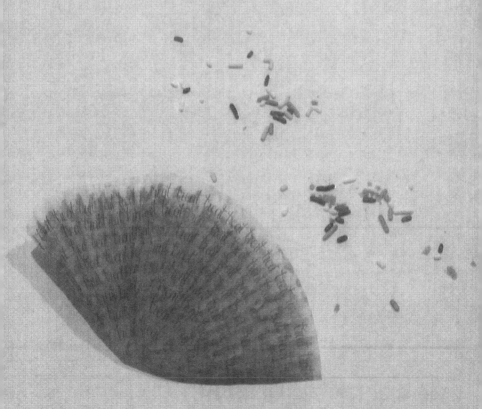

A Normal Kid!

TECH WEEK!
MAY 26TH THROUGH MAY 28TH 2015

Rachel, now 12 years old, was in the ensemble for the middle school play and was at school from 7:20 a.m. until 7:30 p.m., Tuesday through Thursday. She brought no food with her but ate lunch in the school cafeteria and dinner with the cast and crew.

The cast and crew menu was as follows:

- *Tues: pizza & carrots*
- *Wed: several kinds of pasta including one with chicken in a broccoli and cheese sauce, another in a butter sauce and a third with just butter, fruit, cookies for dessert.*
- *Thurs: pizza, salad, fruit, and cookies for dessert*

In case of an emergency, Rachel had her EpiBelt with her that contained Alka Seltzer Gold, Benadryl, and epinephrine. We did not communicate with anyone about *her allergies.* I don't think anyone even knew she had allergies! The director and assistant director had never worked with Rachel before. She used to be a normal kid with food allergies. Now she was just a normal kid who could eat pizza and pasta with cream sauce during tech week. She could go to a cast party without bringing her own snacks or worrying about eating things that may have had cross contact with items to which she was allergic.

We had one happy and tired kid!

5-30-15
Though Rachel appeared to be able to eat most anything, I was wondering what would happen if she ate a whole egg. We never re-did the 3-egg muffin recipe from December, the day Rachel never made it to school because of a major processing episode.

Perhaps I was over analyzing because she was eating egg and cheese sandwiches at school.

Nonetheless, the opportunity to find out arose when Ed took her to the bagel shop for breakfast. She ordered a bacon, egg, and cheese bagel and ate almost all of it. I got a text from my husband: "I'm getting more egg into Rachel!" She also had lunch with her Dad and ordered meatballs with egg noodles.

Nothing happened. Another huge sigh of relief!

5-31-15

It was the beginning of summer and, having rained the night before, it was warm and muggy—a lazy morning. I suggested that we go out for a family breakfast. During our short walk into town I asked everyone what they thought they might want to order. Rachel said, "I'm definitely not getting eggs since I had them yesterday."

Our destination was a popular breakfast place in town that had outdoor seating. Rachel ordered first, as she often did in restaurants. In the past, the preface of her order would have been: "I have food allergies. I'm allergic to eggs, dairy, and mustard. I would like to order a hamburger..." The waitress would need to check the ingredients in the bun to make sure it did not contain eggs or dairy. The grill would need to be cleaned before the burger could be cooked, or the burger would have to be cooked in a clean pan on the grill with a clean spatula. The waitress often needed to go back into the kitchen to talk with the chef before taking the rest of our order. The manager or chef would often have to come out to clarify the allergens. We were always grateful to have direct communication with the kitchen, but our food often took longer to come out than that of other tables.

On this day, we no longer had this stress. Rachel ordered Belgian waffles with chocolate chips and whipped cream on top. My husband and I each ordered an omelet, and our younger daughter ordered scrambled eggs. We ate outside; it rained while we were waiting for our food, but we were safe under the huge table umbrella.

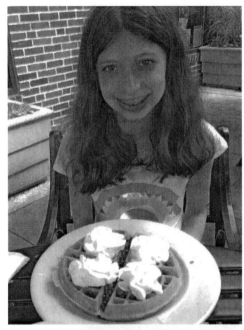

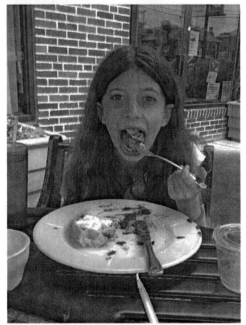

I giggled to myself. Though she had adamantly stated on our walk to the restaurant that she would not be eating eggs for breakfast, she was eating egg in the Belgian waffles.

Did she know? I wondered. Did it matter? No. All that was important was the foods that caused anaphylactic reactions from accidental exposure and cross contact seventeen months ago were confidently being integrated into her diet. And for that I felt eternally grateful to Alexis.

Yet, we were not yet completely out of the woods.

EARLY RELEASE DAY: JUNE 4, 2015
(a small setback)

Rachel's friends walked to the pizza shop for lunch, and afterward the girls walked back to our house to get some money. It was a beautiful late spring afternoon and they wanted to go for ice cream, or in this case frozen custard. I was not worried.

After Rachel came home, she went right to her room. I was in my office doing some work, but I heard her bedroom door slam. I didn't think anything of it. This was a tween-ager, after all. A few minutes later, I went to go check on her. Her back was to me.

"What's the matter?"

When she turned around, I saw how swollen her face and eyes were. "Look," she said.

I immediately gave her two antihistamine that were conveniently located on her dresser; they were still in her room from her recent major processing incident on May 14th.

She said she ordered a kiddie size frozen custard, but they gave her a small and of course she ate the whole thing. As they walked to the toy store, her friend told her that her eyes were red. "I think we should walk back to your house so I can take an Alka Seltzer Gold," she told her friend.

No one ever called me to tell me something was wrong, and she walked home by herself. I was beside myself. She should not have been left alone, especially if she wasn't feeling well. I asked her to call me if this ever happened again. I could have picked her up or contacted another parent to drive her home. Though my daughter was learning how to manage her new found freedom, this incident helped her realize that she needed to learn to manage her allergies. We still had work to do; especially in situations where her allergies began to escalate.

At the same time, I had to work on letting go and I had no issues with her being in town with her friends by herself. But when she did process, she just became my sick baby and that was of course profoundly disturbing.

Success is not linear. Kids must have opportunities to learn and to become independent or they never will. She decided to eat the small size frozen custard instead of a kiddie size. Perhaps she thought nothing of it. Perhaps it was peer pressure to eat what the other kids were eating. Whatever the reason, it was an important lesson in self-control. This was her body, and she needed to learn what was safe.

It didn't upset me that she didn't call me to tell me this was happening before she walked home. It's normal for a child this age to not ask for help. And, again, it's important for them to learn autonomy. But of course as her mother it was hard for me to see her go through the pain. The best I could do was to support her by talking with her about it after the incident.

In the end, this small processing incident was a learning experience for both of us. Rachel was still learning how to handle it as a kid and I as a parent. I was there to teach her that it's OK to try new things and grow, but "with freedom comes responsibility." Teaching your child to make decisions and choices for themselves is not easy, but you cannot do the decision making for them.

I also realized that though we were 17 months into the allergy elimination program, she was still processing, and though Alexis was talking about graduating us, we still had work to do. The issue was not with the frozen custard ingredient list; it was the amount that she had eaten, perhaps combined with having been outside for several hours walking around downtown. Her environmental allergies were far from in balance and her heart rate was probably elevated from walking around with her friends. We needed to go back to gradually increasing amounts of frozen custard to build her tolerance amount from a kiddie size to a small. In any case, she was still able to eat it.

5-29-15

It was almost summer 2015! We were ready to send Rachel to overnight camp, have her graduate from her allergy elimination program, and let her live the rest of her life as a normal and happy tween-ager.

At this point, Rachel was still processing three things: protein isolate in protein bars, the chemicals in frozen yogurt, and undercooked egg in either chocolate mousse or custard-like deserts. Other than that, she was basically eating everything else in normal portion sizes.

As always, I decided to do a little research and contact a friend whose son graduated from Alexis's allergy elimination program six years prior. She said that graduation was a gradual process, but that her son didn't have any problems; he ate everything "but he didn't eat a ton of certain things" as was his preference. Two years after he graduated, they stopped carrying an EpiPen. She did remember one time when her son burned his arm at someone's house. She called the doctor's office and the nurse told her to put raw egg on it. She did, and her son got hives.

Rachel started becoming irresponsible about carrying her EpiBelt with her. Several days during the last week of school she left it in her room, or in the family room at home. How responsible would she be with it at camp, I wondered with minor concern? The camp handled her allergy routine amazingly well last year when we still needed to be vigilant. "Processing" now happened at least an hour after she ate the food in question, so it was still important for Rachel to assume responsibility for herself. She was more likely to step up to the plate without her mother hovering over her.

SENSE OF CLOSURE

Four days before camp started, we had an appointment with Alexis. When the girls came back from camp, we would have three more scheduled appointments, and that would be it. Rachel would graduate from the program! On this day, we talked about portion control. We also talked with Rachel about how to manage any processing issues. We were preparing Rachel for the future. By listening to her body, she could always keep her allergies at bay.

CHAPTER 19

Overnight Camp 2015

MONDAY JUNE 29, 2015
It was the first day of camp, and the girls were sooooo excited to go back.

We left the house at 7 a.m. sharp. Our younger daughter, Iris was jumping out of her skin with excitement! Even though the GPS was completely visible, she must have asked us 100 times "how much longer" until we arrived. Rachel was sitting in the back seat of the car calmly texting her friends. The first year or two there was some sense of anxiety about being away from home without mom and dad for a month, but this was our family's third year and all the girls thought about was seeing their friends.

When we arrived at camp, we were greeted by one of Rachel's counselors. Rachel had this particular counselor in previous years, so she knew about the allergy elimination process and that Rachel would be eating everything this year. Her counselor asked if Rachel still did the tapping and mantra. "Yes, she does," I said. After all, there was a huge mind-body connection; the tapping helped glue this process together.

Before I left, I asked for someone to be "on" Rachel to be sure she was OK with her allergies. I knew once I left the camp, there would be very little information coming from our kids. I wanted to be sure all issues were addressed and that there was a clear process for resolution before we left.

Other than filling out the paperwork, we had no additional communication with the camp director. I just assumed that since Rachel could have her allergy meds in the bunk with her last year, she would also be allowed to have them in the bunk this year. Unfortunately, my assumption was incorrect!

I had packed her probiotics on ice; they were still in the car, as were her inhalers that I would bring to the health center on my way out of the campus. I had stuck one box of Alka Seltzer Gold and one package of antihistamines in with the rest of her sunscreen and other over-the-counter medication just to condense space. It was difficult to get all of their paraphernalia in the car! I realized we had with us FOUR epinephrine auto-injectors and a bunch of loose Alka Seltzer Golds, plus antihistamine chewable tablets. While we were moving in and unpacking, I spoke with the counselor on the front porch of the bunk about Rachel's meds and she told us all medications needed to go through the health center.

Apparently this year the Senior Director didn't like kids carrying their meds around on campus. After negotiation, I agreed with the unit head that I would bring the EpiBelt and all the medication to the health center for approval.

We kissed the girls good-bye and made our last stop at the health center to drop off all the medication. I took two of the four epinephrine devices home, and was told to call the nurse the next day after lunch.

LETTING GO
After lunch on Tuesday afternoon, I spoke with the head nurse to confirm that the medicine situation was under control. The nurse reassured me that Rachel had everything she needed, and I was ready to spend the rest of the month incommunicado with my daughters. Remember, camp policy was that no phone calls were allowed. We could only communicate via letters, snail mail, or scanned PDF documents that were sent to my email account.

I was hoping that this month would help us all take a break from the allergy elimination process but my job as her mother was to keep her safe and so it would be hard to let go.

For one, I would have very little idea of what she was eating at camp. Nor could I ask the special diet chef in the kitchen as he was no longer cooking for her. The camp menu was online, but I had no idea what she actually ate. It was time to let go.

On the other hand, it was a positive thing for Rachel's growth and emotional development. This month at camp, she would have the freedom to choose her meals and snacks without me hovering over her asking her what she ate that day. To allay my constant attention to her diet, I told myself that if she could survive on school cafeteria lunch food for over three months, she could survive on camp dining hall food for one month. Nor did they have whey protein isolates in sports protein bars, the only food now that concerned me.

Nevertheless, I couldn't completely let go of my motherly duty. The campers were going on a day trip where they would be off campus, possibly without medical resources. What type of ice cream would Rachel eat? Would she eat too much? Would she know how to feed herself when given unlimited options? It would be fine, I told myself; we had trained her to be self-sufficient and exercise portion control.

COMMUNICATION FROM CAMP

As expected, we did not receive much communication from our daughters while at camp. The exception was one lame postcard from each daughter that was written on the first day of camp, clearly a forced exercise of the same fill-in-the-blank cards we got every year and which provided little information.

Rachel's postcard told us she was having an amazing time at camp with her friends: "My favorite part of the day was: <u>seeing everyone and being here.</u>" We wanted more specific information, but it looked like my husband and I had to practice self-control!

Parents of kids with food allergies have to learn the balance between letting go and keeping their kids safe. The process that we went through was a balance between solving the problem of Rachel's gut issues and letting go of our lifestyle of living with food allergies. For any parent, sending your kids to camp for a month at a relatively young age is an uneasy emotional process as it's hard to let go of your constant concern for their welfare without your supervision. For us it was doubly so. Fortunately, Rachel is a social, emotionally stable, and well-adjusted kid who was well indoctrinated into the life of a camper.

Still it was hard to be without both of our children for a month. I spent time each morning reading the camp menu options online and looking at pictures from the day before. There was a daily newspaper which included a brief menu for the day. Breakfast menu items included waffles, chocolate chip pancakes, scrambled eggs, hash browns, and French toast. Lunch menu items included pizza, salad, grilled cheese, tomato soup, fries, sliders and sweet potato fries. One day the main lunch was chicken fajitas with rice, beans, salsa, and guacamole. I was sure she would like that.

Dinner options included turkey with homemade mashed potatoes (although I doubt they had dairy because it was a kosher-style camp), BBQ chicken, potatoes, and veggies. Another option was Eggplant Parmesan, BBQ, beef stew with egg noodles, brisket and chicken with veggies. I had no idea exactly what she would be eating every day, or how much! There were always alternate options.

A few days after camp started, the camp's online letter writing system was not working properly. A whole week went by, and there was no news from our daughters. We finally got a letter in the mail from Rachel a week after camp started.

"Dear Mom and Dad,

Sorry it took so long! It's my 3rd day and I can't find my electronic notes that have the barcode on them. They are not where I thought they were. Camp's been great and I'm having a lot of fun...I haven't gotten any letters yet, and I'm almost done with my first book, *Unwanted*. Please Write!!"

Yes, that's my daughter's organizational talent and sense of priority. She couldn't find her stationary and she was most concerned with the book she was reading! It sounded like things were going well. Notice there was no mention in her letter about food.

We got a 2nd letter the next day:

"Dear Mom and Dad,

2 days ago was July 4th. I played games, got popcorn, and (and this part is amazing because I couldn't before) a powdered donut and cookie with milk frosting! I'm on my 3rd book... send me *Hero* 2nd book after *Enchanted*, then *Dearest*..."

Then, just as I was beginning to feel I could breathe easily, on July 9, 2015 at 11:45am (eleven days into the 27-day camp month) I got a call from one of the camp nurses who said "Rachel was rushed in to see the doctor at camp after breakfast because she had a strained neck and they gave her some Tylenol."

Hmmm. A call from the nurse, but... no allergy issues, nothing life threatening. Just a strained muscle. What a relief!

INFORMATION REVEALED
AFTER CAMP PICK-UP

At the end of the month, we picked up the girls. Having witnessed Rachel's progression over the three years she had been a camper, Rachel's counselor was amazed at how she could eat normal food with the rest of the bunk. More than any other counselor, she could appreciate the difference. I asked her if Rachel had ever eaten eggs in the morning. "No, but she ate things with eggs in them like chocolate chip pancakes." Rachel also told me that she ate waffles at camp with homemade heavy whipped cream and strawberry sauce. Yum!

But I learned most of what had transpired from Rachel herself.

INHALER ISSUE

For starters, she told us that during the first week of camp, the nursing staff had misplaced the plastic baggie which contained her inhaler. Furthermore she did not take her long-acting inhaler for 3 nights. On the third night, she was lying in her crowded bunk when one of the counselors noticed she was breathing shallowly and didn't look well. When asked if she was okay, Rachel said, "NO." The counselor walked with Rachel to the health center to find her inhaler and all was resolved.

When she left for camp, her new inhaler had 124 puffs. When she returned home the counter read 99, so she used the long acting inhaler 25 times and she was at camp for 27 days. This indicated that, other than this day she apparently remembered to use her inhaler throughout the rest of the time she was at camp.

EPIPEN ISSUE

If you recall, there was a hoopla at drop off about whether or not she would be allowed to carry her EpiPen with her at camp and I agreed that it would be OK for her to carry only 4 antihistamine and 2 Alka-Seltzer Gold dissolving tablets. However, at pick-up I found out they also gave her an EpiPen to carry in her EpiBelt. After I picked her up, the EpiPen was in her EpiBelt and she told me the director had a conversation with her about making sure she would be responsible.

What was going on?

More conversation came out in the car on the way home. The girls explained that Rachel had visited her sister's bunk on a rainy day and left her polka-dot Epibelt there by accident. Apparently, she took it off and it then fell under the bunk bed where it was found a few days later. Rachel told someone in her bunk about its mysterious disappearance and the counselors helped her find it. Fortunately, nothing happened during this time but if something had, she was always able to go to the health center. No one bothered to mention this in any of the camp letters, so I had no idea.

MINOR INCIDENTS
Rachel told me there were a few times when she used her meds. She had some milk and cookies for dessert during dinner one night, her lips became a little swollen, and her throat felt a little tight. She visited the nurse to take an "Alka" and that was it. When she told me, I was proud of her for exhibiting responsibility and unconcerned about the incident since it was so minor. I did not receive any phone calls about this since I signed a release.

I also learned that Rachel had a lot of ice cream at the banquet on the last night of camp. Apparently her eyes started to itch and she had a few hives on one of her arms. She went to the health center and took two chewable tablets of Benadryl. She confessed she also wanted to take the Benadryl partly because she wanted to go to sleep as Benedryl makes you sleepy. In the end, though her symptoms weren't bad, she behaved responsibly, and I was proud that she was learning how to take care of herself.

AT HOME AND DOING GREAT

On her first night home, she had a Babybel cheese for a snack and ice cream for dessert. She scooped the ice cream herself – as much as she wanted. No problems.

The rest of the summer was amazing! When the girls got home from camp, we spent some time at Grandma's house in New Jersey. Rachel got a new pocketbook from Grandma, named "G." She used it to carry her epi, antihistamine, and Alka tablets for precautionary purposes.

VERMONT VACATION

At the end of the summer, we had a two-week vacation in Vermont. Ed and I were able to either work during the day or go hiking. The girls went to a resort day camp where Rachel once again could eat the camp lunch and ice cream. At night, we spent time together as a family.

As Rachel was old enough to leave camp on her own at the end of the day, I taught her how to charge items to the room. Most days, we gave her the privilege of going to the on-campus Ben & Jerry's store after camp with her friends, where she could charge the creamy cold goodies to our account. Her favorite flavor was Cherry Garcia. I was so excited that Rachel could eat ice cream in Ben and Jerry's home state!

One night she enjoyed a cheeseburger at Gracie's restaurant and a Vermont maple creemee, (Vermont's version of soft-serve ice cream) in Stowe after dinner. We worked hard to get to this point, so we talked about what Rachel's rewards might be for completing the allergy elimination program. Some ideas were horseback riding lessons or voice lessons. Rachel really wanted a family dog. We were working on this one, but it didn't seem likely because of my younger daughter and husband's environmental allergies.

So we tried for all three reward options. Rachel first opted for horseback riding lessons, which she took for a few months, but then she didn't like the teacher, so she stopped. This was after I spent lots of money on new riding boots and the tight fitting trousers with leather patches on the inside of the knees to match. Once school commenced in September, she started taking voice lessons which she loved and continued for several years. She has such a beautiful voice!

However, we never did get that family dog. We tried going to a poodle breeder one sunny fall afternoon, but after spending more than an hour in the breeder's family room, Ed was practically wheezing, and Iris' eyes were so red and itchy that we decided to forgo the idea. Perhaps we solved the issues of Rachel's food allergies, but we were not yet finished with the rest of the allergy issues in our family.

MINOR PROCESSING

We were almost 100% clear of any food allergy issues, but not quite. Before Labor Day, I made eggplant soaked in an egg wash and baked with breadcrumbs and cheese. I was trying to hurry the dish; for some reason, I took it out of the oven too soon. It turned out to be undercooked, and it made Rachel feel sick. This could happen to anyone. She didn't have an allergic reaction, she just felt sick, but she knows her body so well because she had so many reactions in her life that she could pinpoint what it was. Plus I knew I had taken it out of the oven a little too soon. I gave her some antihistamine before bed and she was fine.

CHAPTER 20

A New Year, 2015

FORMS! FORMS! FORMS! A week after her first day of seventh grade, I called the school nurse to give her a heads up that I would be stopping by with Rachel's emergency meds and her medical forms. I dreaded this visit, expecting to meet with yet another bureaucratic medical office. Unfortunately, my expectations were realized.

First, the nurse wouldn't accept the doctor's health memorandum form because it would expire in April. She asked me to go back to the doctor and get a new form signed that would last the whole year. I explained that I would not go to the doctor just to get a revised signature. Then the nurse would not accept the note from the doctor that allowed her to take Alka-Seltzer Gold because it was signed in January and would expire after one year.

The nurse also could not accept the EpiPen because it didn't have the pharmacy label on it. I decided to take it home with me because it was the only EpiPen we had that had not yet expired. Rachel had carried one with her since she was ten years old, but the nurse's office also had a stock supply. We learned this on the last day of second grade when Rachel was "epied" by the nurse and taken to the hospital in an ambulance. Then the nurse didn't want Rachel's antihistamine because she said they had gallons of the liquid kind in their office.

The nurse explained that the food services department had instructions not to allow her to eat anything that she was allergic to at school. That was interesting because she had been buying lunch every day in the 6th grade since March and every day dur-ing the first week of 7th grade without any problems. The nurse explained that this was a very gray area. I understood.

Then the nurse asked me to fill out six forms: two forms for each of the medications that she would be allowed to carry at school for emergency purposes. I needed to fill out one form for the state and one for the school for each medication. That meant two forms each for EpiPen, inhaler, and Alka-Seltzer Gold. I had to complete and sign six forms just in case she might need these medications!

I asked if I could consolidate the medical forms. She thought I was kidding. I left the forms and the Alka-Seltzer Gold in the nurse's office and escaped bureaucracy by walking out to my car in the 95 degree, post Labor Day heat.

The next morning I informed Rachel that I took care of all the nurse forms so she wouldn't have to worry and that I filled out the necessary forms in case she needed to take any medication. Her comment: "So if I need to save my life, I can." I said "Yes," What a wit my daughter has!

I replaced the expired EpiPen Rachel was carrying in her purse with the unexpired one that I decided not to leave with the nurse. It made more sense for Rachel to have it with her at all times than for it to be in the nurse's office since she was now going out for ice cream with her friends on the way home from school. Plus she could carry it with her when the kids went on field trips.

I didn't expect anything to happen at this point. I knew Rachel would take an Alka or antihistamine on her own if she needed it. But if she were in a panicked state from having difficulty breathing, she might not be able to administer the EpiPen; it was important to keep it available so an adult could quickly intervene.

ROSH HASHANAH, SEPTEMBER 2015
Rosh Hashanah is the beginning of a ten-day period of prayer, self-examination and repentance known as the Days of Awe or the High Holy Days that Jews observe throughout the world.

Along with the religious observance are traditional homemade recipes. One is noodle kugel made with egg. I made this yummy dish the Friday before Rosh Hashanah – our first year that I didn't have to substitute the eggs! It was not only fun to have a traditional kugel, but it remained a necessary part of the desensitization process for Rachel to eat eggs.

The recipe called for six eggs, butter, cottage cheese, sour cream and milk. That night, Rachel ate a very small piece of the kugel and had no processing issues. What an accomplishment after all the difficulty in getting her to eat eggs.

During dinner that night, we discussed my famous squash soufflé. Rachel made it clear that she hated when I made it with eggs as I had during Passover. I didn't tell her that the noodle kugel also had six eggs in its recipe, nor did I mention that the noodles themselves were made with eggs.

DAMAGED PROTEIN
However, I was prematurely excited. Two days later, during Erev Rosh Hashanah dinner, Rachel wouldn't even put the noodle kugel on her plate! Instead, she and her sister talked about how the kugel they ate at camp was much better and sweeter than the one I made. Hmmm, I thought, I'm going to have to get that camp recipe. And I would on mother/daughter weekend the following April. (See Appendix E)

That same night, we had an unexpected incident that led me to discover the possible underlying cause of some of her mysterious processing incidents.

Once we finished dinner, Rachel ate a full serving of frozen yogurt. As we headed to Temple for the Erev Rosh Hashanah service, she started blowing her nose, "I think I need to take an Alka," she said quietly to her Dad as they walked into the Temple. I was a few steps behind with her younger sister, so I didn't hear.

At 8:00 p.m. when I got to the doors of the sanctuary, my daughter was in the ladies room. My husband told me "She went to take an Alka". I was glad she took charge of the situation – a step in the right direction – but of course I went to check on her. She told me she couldn't figure out how to take an Alka in the bathroom, so she took four antihistamine tablets.

"Four. Really?" It was the full adult dose, which seemed like a lot to me. I normally gave her two chewable antihistamine tablets that amounted to half the adult dose. I noticed that she had "eye epaulets" in the inside corners of her eyes, meaning that her sphenoid and ethmoid sinuses were swollen.

She had little bumps in between her nose and both tear ducts. This was a sign of processing and usually led to more swelling of the sinuses. I tried to keep my cool as we were in Temple for the commencement of the High Holy days. It is said that "on Rosh Hashanah it is written and on Yom Kippur it is sealed." Could the energy of the universe be coming into play? I hoped not.

All four of us sat at the back of the sanctuary, but Rachel kept getting up to walk out so she could blow her nose. Her eyes were now completely swollen. Ed told me to "go out there with her". This was real; I was no longer overreacting!

Rachel and I sat on the couch outside of the sanctuary listening to the beautifully sung musical prayers that were so familiar and comforting to both of us. Rachel did her mantra and tapping. I joined her, and then we just sat there. I wrapped my arm around her, and we talked about why this might be happening. Rachel thought she might have reacted because the frozen yogurt was melted. I doubted this was true. I thought it might have been the egg and dairy combination, the chemicals, or both combined.

At 8:30 p.m. Rachel said she felt worse than she did before she took the antihistamine. My husband and my other daughter came out of the sanctuary to check on us. Ed walked to the car, picked us up, and drove us home. I looked at the label of the frozen yogurt. It contained egg yolks. I did not see how much frozen yogurt was in the bowl before we left, but my husband said he thought it was a lot and at the time he had told her to stop scooping. Ed hypothesized that, though she had developed a tolerance, her issues were not entirely over.

At 9:00 p.m. the antihistamine was making Rachel tired, so she went to bed. I told her "this just means you will need to eat more frozen yogurt." She smiled at that and fell asleep.

The next morning Rachel slept much later than normal. Her dad had a conversation with her about how important it was to continue to eat the things she worked so hard to be able to eat so she didn't lose the tolerance. We were not sure how much she understood what we were saying, but she did eat a smaller amount of the frozen yogurt the next day and nothing happened.

Two days later she had chicken soup for dinner with matzo balls and egg noodles. I know that she ate 66% of an egg in the matzo balls because I made them from scratch. I have no idea how much the egg noodles added to this equation, but she was once again fine. No processing. Totally normal. Still, I was wracking my brains on how to get her to eat more egg and trying to figure out what caused the problem.

PROTEINS
Why could Rachel eat cheese sticks and pizza, but she had trouble with sports bars? Similar to this, why was it she could now eat ice cream, but she had trouble with the same brand of frozen yogurt?

I decided to do some research on the nutritional benefits of frozen yogurt. I learned that the egg content may not have been what caused Rachel's processing. Rather, the damaged proteins in processed foods may have been the culprit. Kia Sanford, a clinical nutritionist counselor has a video on aol.com entitled "The truth about frozen yogurt and ice cream" in which she discusses the dairy industry. She states,

"When you start taking fat out of a dairy product, you have to put something in it to give what's called in the industry, 'mouthfeel' which is what makes it feel creamy and satisfying in your mouth. Therefore the sugar content increases. This makes frozen yogurt a lot higher in sugar. It may be lower in fat, but you end up with more of the damaged proteins because of the way that fat is pulled out of milk."

Interesting! Sugar helps the frozen yogurt feel better in your mouth but along with it comes damaged proteins.

This led me to believe that perhaps Rachel's body had rejected processed food because of the damaged proteins rather than protein in eggs or dairy. This may also have been why she had an allergic reaction to the whey protein isolate, the last ingredient in the peanut butter that she ate in October 2012 before we started this desensitization process. It may also have been damaged protein.

Much research has pointed to the fact that processing changes the way foods are digested and assimilated in our bodies. New evidence is mounting daily that processed foods also contribute to an imbalanced inner ecosystem; beneficial microflora cannot survive in a digestive tract over-run by toxic bacteria from the chemicals used to provide texture, flavor and color (and not always listed on labels), along with the hormones and antibiotics added to the food supply. Altering proteins can change metabolism patterns which in turn can contribute to the overall allergic nature of any given protein. (See Appendix C)

How can we all eat more whole food? In Appendix D, I have listed companies that are ditching artificial ingredients for whole food ingredients. As a rule of thumb, try to eat whole, real food in place of processed food. Load up your menu with fresh fruits and veggies – organic is always best -- healthy grains, lentils, nuts, seeds and grass fed beef if you wish to eat meat.

9-18-15
After school, Rachel dropped off her backpack and rode back into town to get some ice cream with her friends. At 3:30, I called her friend's mother who said they were hang-ing out in town, and I texted Rachel to find out where she was. She texted back, "Going home. All my friends are coming."

The next thing I knew, five twelve-year-olds who had just eaten ice cream and ridden their bikes from the center of town to our house were sitting on the family room couch and watching a video on someone's iPad. There was an excited energy, the same as you would expect anywhere with a bunch of tweens exploring their independence. Everything was fine, except that my daughter's voice was slightly raspy when she spoke.

I asked if anyone wanted a glass of water, hoping that Rachel would use the opportunity to take an Alka if she thought she needed one. Since it was a hot sticky day, everyone took a cup from the cabinet and helped themselves to a cup of water. Rachel did not take me up on the 'Alka' opportunity. She was too 'cool' to be bothered with complying with a motherly request in front of her friends and doing so would embarrass her. I let it go. She was fine.

Subsequently I found out which place the kids went to for ice cream and later that week, went to the ice cream store to check the ingredients. There was no egg in the ice cream, but there were a lot of chemicals. Rachel and I talked about how her voice was raspy after eating the ice cream and that there was no egg in the ice cream.

I asked her how much she ate, and she said it was a normal size. She also said that she didn't finish the whole thing. I surmised that her raspy throat was from the volume of artificial chemicals. She would have to continue eating different types of ice cream for her body to get used to tolerating them. The important thing was that Rachel was able to enjoy a Friday afternoon with her friends and be a part of the ice cream-eating crowd instead of having to eat a dairy-free cupcake like she used to before we started this program.

9-25-15
A week later, Rachel was eating anything she wanted. She had a bowl of the same frozen yogurt treat for a snack after school and approximately 60% of an egg in her matzo ball soup for dinner without any processing.

I decided to circle back with Alexis this week to ask if these ongoing issues with tolerance were normal. I asked her about both the frozen yogurt and the ice cream with chemical ingredients added. She said this sometimes happens, and she reminded me that we had trouble with ice cream and frozen yogurt in the past. She asked if we wanted to come in for a visit but I declined. So long as Alexis was aware of the incident and was confident that everything would be OK, I was satisfied. I knew she was there for us if we needed her, but we would continue to work on this on our own.

I also told Alexis it was so difficult to get Rachel to eat egg. She suggested buying fresh egg pasta at Whole Foods, which I did. The following Saturday I gave it to Rachel for lunch with some organic butter. She ate it and nothing happened.

10-4-15
On Sunday morning, Rachel said the chocolate zucchini bread or challah that we often ate for breakfast made her throat get tight, but "when I drink water it goes away." The chocolate zucchini bread and challah were both made with organic eggs. I was uncertain what was going on.

We had a nice conversation about eating fruits and veggies to stay healthy, as I was concerned about the poor quality of the school lunch food that she had been eating without problems, at least so far this year – basically a lot of pizza and meatball subs (which I'm sure were highly processed and laden with chemicals and antibiotics) while passing up salad, apples and carrots because of her braces. Since she had more time to eat meals and snacks at home where I could cut up the items into smaller pieces, she would eat more fruits and veggies and a more balanced diet at home.

We talked about her health, but I was still happy that she had the freedom to make these choices.

In the afternoon, she scooped her own bowl of frozen yogurt. A couple hours later, she went up in her room to lie in her bed, feeling tired. I asked her if she wanted an Alka and she said "No. It's not that." She said her stomach hurt, that it had been hurting all day, and that she just didn't feel well. Her eyes weren't swollen in an allergic kind of way, but they were watery. Maybe she was just coming down with something. I gave her a sip of some plain water and hoped she would sleep.

But instead she got up, went downstairs and ate some guacamole with plain crackers. She blew her nose again and said her stomach hurt a little. It had been three hours since she had eaten the frozen yogurt. It occurred to me that my younger daughter had been sneezing all weekend. I had never stopped to analyze how often or with what frequency this was occurring with my other daughter. I concluded that perhaps Rachel and Iris were both fighting a cold or some other virus. There was so much to let go of. I had to learn that not everything was an allergic reaction. Sometimes kids just get sick! This virus lasted the normal cycle of about a week.

WORKING ON FROZEN YOGURT: 10-25-15

A few weeks later, a similar scene occurred. In the afternoon, I filled an eight-ounce ramekin with frozen yogurt and fancied it up, putting a little more whipped cream on top, then we made a video of me dispensing whipped cream into Rachel's mouth. She ate it. Nothing happened.

A little later, Rachel was hungry. Since it was before dinner, she decided to have some protein to fill her and ate a cheese stick.

Soon after, she was lying on her bed complaining that her stomach hurt and looked like she was in pain. Immediately, I thought it might be processing and I gave her two Alkas. But my wise daughter said it couldn't be the frozen yogurt because that was two hours ago and she did not have any of the usual symptoms. Her nose was not running, and there was no flushing, puffy eyes, or hives – just a stomach ache. She thought it might be growing pains. I was under the assumption that growing pains happened in your legs! But still, she was right. My daughter had an amazing sense of her body for a twelve year old, and I was so proud of her!

Though I didn't know why she had pains in her stomach, as long as she wasn't showing any signs of allergic reaction I wasn't worried.

The rest of the evening was perfectly normal. For dinner she ate half an avocado, Trader Joe's stuffed chicken breast with cranberry apple stuffing, sweet potato fries, and edamame (soy). At 7 p.m. she went over a friend's house for her robotics team meeting.

A few days later, she ate some frozen yogurt for dessert right out of the carton. Nothing happened. Nor did anything happen the next day when I gave her an 8oz. ramekin filled with frozen yogurt and topped with whipped cream.

Amazing! What a journey we went through.

HALLOWEEN!: 10-31-15
I started out this journey talking about how in 2015, my Rachel ate chocolate to her heart's delight at Halloween and how I didn't even feel the need to go trick or treating with my daughters to assure Rachel didn't eat anything that would cause an allergic reaction. In fact, I was so confident that she could eat whatever she pleased that I permitted her Halloween adventure to include a five-girl sleepover at her friend's house even though I wouldn't see her until the next morning!

Since we had time on Saturday morning before the Halloween festivities began, I suggested that Rachel eat a serving of the frozen yogurt at 11:00 a.m., so long as she ate her orange or some fruits and veggies first. She was delighted that I would suggest she eat sugar in the morning on the same day that she was expecting to eat lots of candy later in the evening! She took out the pint size carton, let it melt a little, and put her portion into a large cereal bowl. I did not see how much she portioned out in-to the bowl or how much she ate. She took as much as she wanted and then said. "I'm done. I just don't want anymore," and put the rest in the freezer. Nothing happened.

At 1:15 she had a portion of Buitoni Spinach Cheese Tortellini mixed with frozen peas and tomato sauce for lunch. This pasta contained eggs and was filled with ricotta, parmesan and Romano cheeses. Nothing happened.

The next morning, after I picked her up from the sleepover, I asked Rachel how much candy she ate. "Not much; only about ten pieces." She ate candy and nothing happened. Yeah for us!

At dinner, I gave Rachel a baked potato with butter and sour cream. She said "This is making my stomach feel sick." I told her not to eat anymore; Ed suggested that she take some Alka, which she did. We wondered why she could eat frozen yogurt and pizza but she was now having an issue with the sour cream and butter on her potato.

Then she told me she felt the same sickness when she ate KitKat and Crunch bars, but *not* when she ate Swedish Fish, Dots, Junior Mints, or Whoppers. How could this be? Why can she eat three slices of pizza with no problem, a full portion of cheese tortellini with no problem, but then eat a small Halloween fun size candy bar and feel sick? What was in the sour cream and butter that made her sick? I didn't know what to make of this. But again, I assumed the answer lay in the different added chemicals.

11-2-15

When Rachel came home from school, her eyes were watering. She had been dizzy and tired before lunch, so she went to the nurse and lay down for about 10 minutes. At lunch, she ate a cheeseburger on a bun with carrots, a whole wheat Rice Crispy Treat, and half a cupcake that her friend gave her.

Ten minutes after lunch she started feeling the tightness in her throat. She asked the substitute teacher if she could go to her locker to take an Alka, which he allowed. Rachel put 2 Alkas into a bottle of water and spilled a little, so she said she had about 1 ½ dissolved fizzy tablets.

I wondered why this happened at school and made an appointment to see Alexis the next day.

11-3-15

After testing her with her electro-dermal device, Alexis said there was a lot of stuff in Rachel's energy field, including strep and a lot of viruses. She told me to take Rachel to the doctor to get a strep test. If she had strep, she would need to get treated with an antibiotic to clear it up.

I took her to the pediatrician that same day and, fortunately the strep test was negative. "Sometimes kids have stomach aches," Dr. Jacqui said.

I told her that the school wanted an updated allergy action plan and updated note allowing the nursing staff to give her an Alka if necessary.

She asked me why we needed an allergy action plan if Rachel was eating everything. I explained, "Because we weren't re-tested." She said she wouldn't give Rachel an allergy test because she was already eating everything and that test results weren't always accurate. She felt that if Rachel is eating dairy, her processing/reactions were from something else.

I was extremely relieved. Neither the pediatrician nor Alexis were concerned about the tightness in her throat.

The pediatrician removed the allergens from the allergy action plan and gave me the revised blank allergy action plan and an updated Alka note. Then she offered me the option of giving it to the school nurse now or waiting until next April. I have so much respect for our pediatrician! She made me feel validated.

SCHOOL LUNCH: MARCH 21, 2016, FIRST DAY OF SPRING

As I have repeatedly mentioned, I felt obligated to give Rachel processed food so her body could get used to the chemicals even though I had learned how damaging eating this food is for all of our health. What could I do to get her to eat more healthily? Well, as it turned out the answer was to let Rachel's own wisdom shine through.

In the spring, I received an email from the public school food service accounting department explaining that Rachel owed forty cents on her lunch account. I wondered how she could have gone through so much money in her account when I had recently put in a substantial sum.

I called Rachel into my office to ask her to look at her on line account with me. Her eyes welled up with tears. "You didn't do anything wrong," I said. "I'm just trying to figure out how you could have gone through so much money in such a short period of time."

"I know," she said. "It's just that when I had food allergies, I used to eat healthy food, then when I didn't have them anymore, it was exciting to be able to eat in the school cafeteria. But I hate the food there!" It turned out that the novelty of eating food in the school cafeteria wore off. A year prior, her friends were mesmerized that Rachel could even eat the lunches that were made in the school cafeteria. She was excited to be part of the peer group, but now it wasn't fun anymore.

But why was the amount of money she spent double on some days? As it turned out, on the days that they had food that she liked, like pizza and quesadillas, she would buy two. On the other days, for example taco day when they had the "mystery meat" she bought just one main lunch. However, for the most part she didn't like the food, so I happily agreed to get up a little earlier to make her lunch in the mornings.

The first day I made her wontons from Costco and put them in a thermos for her main lunch then added some fruits and veggies to for a side dish. The second day, I made her a tuna sandwich along with an orange, individual serving of guacamole and some organic blue corn chips. The third day I filled a thermos with Italian Wedding Soup (See Appendix E).

For an extra ounce of love, I added a milk chocolate kiss.

No processing.

YOUTH GROUP CHOCOLATE SEDER: APRIL 29, 2016

If you are a kid with a dairy allergy, it's hard to eat conventional chocolate which tends to be made with milk. Once Rachel could eat dairy, eating chocolate was a huge treat. And so what could be more exciting than a Chocolate Seder given by our Temple Youth Group. "The Seder will include Matzah Ball soup, as well as lots of different kinds of chocolate - chocolate milk, chocolate matzah, dark chocolate, milk chocolate, white chocolate, and more. All products will be nut-free and there will be dairy-free options as well. When you check in with our staff, we'll verify both the emergency contact information and any allergies or dietary needs that you provided during registration."

Two years ago, we might not even have signed her up for this fun youth group event, but now I was excited for Rachel because I knew she would enjoy it. I was completely unconcerned that she would have egg in the matzo ball soup and then milk chocolate immediately after.

RACHEL'S BAT MITZVAH: JUNE 4, 2016

On June 4, 2016, Rachel had her Bat Mitzvah, something we had been planning for years. This event was the celebration of Rachel's coming of age and her graduation from food allergy issues so it was spectacular in every way!

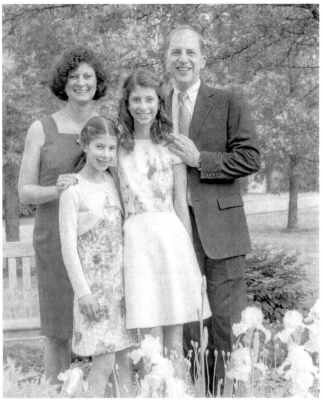

Holli, Iris, Rachel and Ed June 4, 2016

Rachel felt being in the mountains connected her more with God, so at Rachel's request, we held her Bat Mitzvah service at a small Synagogue in Stowe, VT. Then we had a huge celebration a few miles away at Smuggler's Notch, our favorite family vacation resort.

The Bat Mitzvah was fabulous! Over the top! One hundred of our closest friends and relatives spent the entire weekend eating in celebration with us. We had four different food related events throughout the weekend, plus an afternoon pool party and sleepover for Rachel and her friends.

In the end, Rachel ate cake from Mirabella's in Burlington made with REAL BUTTERCREAM!, chocolate mousse, chocolate cake, ice cream, brownies, mozzarella sticks, and Old Homestead farms beef burger with Cabot cheddar cheese. She wouldn't however eat the deviled eggs. At the luncheon on Saturday afternoon she squealed, "Why are there eggs at my Bat Mitzvah!" We had no concerns about allergies, yet her taste buds had distinct preferences.

Ed and I beamed throughout the entire weekend. Rachel did a magnificent job leading the entire service on Saturday along with Rabbi David. Here are some excerpts:

Her Torah portion was about respecting the environment.

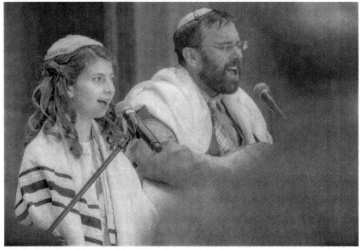

Rachel and Rabbi David in Vermont

"...when we respect the environment, we are rewarded, but when we destroy or hurt the environment, bad things will happen. The environment is essential... trees represent life, they create oxygen, they help humans live, and therefore we need to protect them. Although we might not recognize it, when we respect the environment, all of humanity will be rewarded.

This relates to my Torah portion, because I'm taking part in saving and protecting the environment. My mom always tells me that "with freedom comes responsibility". My Torah portion teaches that we have a responsibility to the land. With this freedom and responsibility, I will continue to find ways to help the environment and keep the earth clean."

Rachel was so well prepared that soon after her bat mitzvah she received a letter from our Cantor asking her to chant Haftora at our synagogue in Boston on Yom Kippur, our most holy holiday. On October 12, 2016 over 1,000 people who attended the service were blessed with hearing our daughter's beautiful voice.

Concluding Notes

I wanted to write this book because I felt compelled to tell my story to the whole world in the hope of inspiring others to try new approaches to health issues. In this way, our story of redemption may be the stepping stone for others to seek alternative treatments that marry Eastern and Western philosophies of health. Had we not combined both approaches, I don't know if we would have been as successful in healing Rachel of life-threatening allergies to egg, dairy and mustard.

While training the body's immune system to work properly by developing tolerance to a harmless protein has been used in Western medicine, Alexis's use of the electro-dermal "energy" device comes from modern technology. Her experience with other techniques, including the mind/body "holistic" component comes from Eastern philosophy, something Western medicine virtually ignores.

Further, until more recently Western medicine has been ignoring the importance of the microbiome and the need for probiotics; recall that taking a daily probiotic was an essential part of Rachel's therapy. But this too is now changing as new research comes out daily about how poor gut flora is the underlying cause for much illness and mental health issues. In fact, Western doctors are now doing a procedure called Fecal Microbiota Transplant (FMT) in which stool is collected from a tested donor, mixed with a saline or other solution, strained, and placed in a patient, by colonoscopy, endoscopy, sigmoidoscopy, or enema for the purpose of treating recurrent *C. difficile colitis*. This is also now being used in trials to treat food allergy patients.

It still amazes and astonishes me that after more than a decade of living without the food she was once allergic to, my daughter will now ask me to buy Babybel cheese at the supermarket because she loves it! She will go to Costco with my husband, have a tasting of Boursin cheese and then insist that they purchase the entire three bulk pack. She can now eat ice cream and pizza with her friends, at a birthday party or anytime.

We can fly on an airplane without bringing any food with us and not have to worry about cross-contamination issues. She can go to a buffet at a party and taste all of the fancy cakes. She can go out to dinner with her grandparents, order French onion soup for an appetizer, and have a cheddar burger for her main entree. We can go out for breakfast as a family and share waffles and pancakes, and she can go to overnight camp without having a special diet or eating specially prepared foods. It is my hope that the systematic desensitization method we used becomes the wave of the future.

I learned so much from this journey. If my daughter was not born with her food allergies, I never would have really understood the full extent to which our planet is in trouble because of the food we consider "normal." I believe that food allergies can be fixed along with our food supply and our environment if we learn to eat whole food in place of processed food. The time to make this change is now. I'm hoping that reading this book will empower people to make these changes.

I know everyone can make a difference. This book is just one story that documents how changes can be made and the huge difference it made in our lives. I encourage the medical community to embrace the health coaching community and vice versa; via functional medicine, traditional medicine can learn from Eastern concepts of energy, the use of the electro-dermal device, and the mind/body connection. It may not be easy, but I think it speaks to the future of healthcare in our country.

Again, I caution the reader to not try this method on your own at home without the proper help, support, and guidance of an advanced health coach practitioner properly trained to do the work that supports this method.

We've truly gone From *Anaphylaxis to Butter Cream!*

Appendices

Below are two appendices of the food Rachel ate: as an infant, and on a trip to visit family when she was eight. Free of eggs, milk, dairy and mustard, the foods to which she was allergic, these foods were deemed safe to eat by the allergist and nutritionist. However, they were unhealthy! Though I didn't know it at the time, they were non-organic. These foods also contained much gluten which allows foreign particles to enter into the digestive system, as well as chemicals, hormones, antibiotics and other synthetic ingredients, all of which are hard to digest and assimilate. All this adds up to bad food, and I later learned that this was further deteriorating Rachel's immune system. But at this time, I was uneducated about healthy eating; my main concern was that Rachel avoid all foods to which she was allergic.

Appendix A
Sample of Rachel's Diet at One Year Old

Day 1:
Breakfast: Pasta (durum and Jerusalem artichokes) and tuna. First baby food jar : carrot, beef and barley. Second baby food jar : prunes and apples

Lunch: Browned hamburger meat, the rest of the prunes, pasta, green peas

Snack: Rice cakes and apple

Dinner: Apple, whole wheat pasta, tuna

Day 2:
Breakfast: Puffins cereal (corn mix): she didn't like it and ate very little. Beechnut turkey rice dinner, sweet potatoes, turkey, rice, carrots, peas (a few bites), apple, a few bites, plain rice cake, plain matzo

Lunch: Hamburger, mixed veggies (frozen) peas, peaches, a few bites of apple

Snack: Apple, Lender's plain frozen bagel

Dinner: Peas whole wheat pasta, browned ground beef

Day 3:
Breakfast: Pasta, a little beef, cinnamon apple granola and peaches

Lunch: Fish sticks, peas, and pasta

Snack: Rice Cake and apple

Dinner: Some ground beef, and peaches, turkey, rice baby food

Day 4:
Breakfast: Pasta, beef, apricots/mixed fruit

Lunch: A small amount of ground beef, 3 bites of prunes, apricot and whole pear, peas, 2 fish sticks, pasta, apple cinnamon rice cake

Snack: Snap pea crisps and Nabisco graham crackers

Dinner: Tuna steak, country veggies and brown rice, whole wheat and regular pasta mixed together

Appendix B
April 2011: Instructions for Rachel's Trip to Pittsburgh to Visit Family

Rachel's normal breakfast is a Luna bar.

For lunch, she usually has a sandwich or soy yogurt (but some soy yogurts have whey, casein, or other dairy products), some fruit, and something else. She also likes roast beef lunch meat (without any bread or anything else), but she is currently a little sick of it. We can send some high fiber fruit leather snacks that she likes from Trader Joe's.

For dinner, hamburger or chicken nuggets either from Costco (Kirkland, shaped like Mickey Mouse) or Empire. She eats carrots, beans (black eyed peas from a can), and some other veggies (see below).

Fiber One hamburger buns and bread are staples in our house to get the fiber into Rachel. (We'll also send along some Fiber Gummies, but those are just a weak sup-plement. Her diet is key.)

Below are some foods that she eats and likes. Morning snack is often snap-pea crisps or something similar. Afternoon snack is variable, but often "an appetizer" of carrots or some similar healthy food around 4:30.

WHAT'S OUT?
Eggs, dairy, mustard, and kamut flour. Garlic is borderline. She can usually tolerate a little garlic, but be careful.

WHAT'S IN?
Almonds and peanuts. Yea!!!! She should really have some form of each at least 3 times a week to keep the allergy from returning.

Baked sweet potato with pareve margarine.

Mango, blackberries, cantaloupe, oranges, and apples.
Celery with almond/peanut butter and raisins (ants on a log).

Hamburger. Always make sure that it's a pure beef burger, 100% cow. Egg is an obvious issue, but lots of pre-made burgers have mustard in them.

Carrots, edamame, and asparagus, steamed plain.

Boiled artichoke ~45 mins, completely plain.

Silk soy yogurt: peach, strawberry, banana. There are other brands of soy yogurt, but some have dairy ingredients. Stay away from Stonyfield Farm. It's got casein.

Either Tofutti cuties or SO delicious Neapolitan mini ice cream sandwiches are her desserts every night.

Tuna: plain (maybe w/lemon).

Butternut squash mashed with pareve margarine and brown sugar.

Vegan American Flavor Galaxy Nutritional Foods soy vegan cheese slices.

Appendix C
New Findings

Being a food allergy coach is my passion and life's work. As such, I make every attempt to stay informed. Herewith is some new information I learned while I wrote Rachel's diary.

PEANUT PATCH: <u>ANOTHER PROMISE TO END PEANUT ALLERGY</u> – YAHOO HEALTH

"Dr. Pierre-Henri Benhamou of DBV Technologies, a publicly traded French bio-pharmaceutical company, has created Viaskin Peanut, a patch worn by those afflicted and changed daily. The patch works by slowly releasing small amounts of peanut protein onto the skin. According to the company, while the immune system would normally reject the protein in higher doses with deadly consequences, the patch slowly builds a tolerance supposedly resulting in complete desensitization."

I found some problems with the notion of a patch. As far as I knew, this method was not first taking into account the importance of balancing the immune system or resetting the microbiome, and I was sure it was not using energy techniques to heal the underlying emotional issues. I was concerned that the peanut patch was a drug. Nevertheless, it would be interesting to see the long term effects of this patch. Further, if it proves useful, the patch may lead to a treatment for multiple food allergies. As of the writing of this book, Viaskin was conducting clinical trials for peanut, milk, and egg.

The company was also working on technology platforms for immunology and vaccines. All of these treatments were still new and none had implemented procedures in place.

EGG ALLERGY

In July 2012, *The New England Journal of Medicine* published a study on an oral immunotherapy for treatment of egg allergy in children: "Allergy solutions take new form." Using a small sample, 1/3 of the children were cured. The study did not address the issue of the immune system in the gut.

NEW LEAP STUDY

In March 2015 there was a lot of news press about the completed "LEAP" study that claimed the same evidence that was noted in Britain in 2008, namely that consumption of peanuts in infancy is associated with a low evidence of peanut allergies.

MORE DOCTORS GETTING ON BOARD
An ABC news clip, "Utah Doctor 'frees' Children from Isolating Food Allergies," stated that Dr. Douglas Jones of Rocky Mountain Allergy, Asthma, and Immunology successfully treated more than 50 patients with OIT.

SOME DISAPPOINTING FINDINGS
DAIRY AND ORAL IMMUNOTHERAPY
Allergic Living published an article in March 2013 from the 2013 AAAAI Allergists' Conference discussing findings that showed that desensitization wasn't holding up for dairy allergy patients who were having frequent symptoms three to five years after the trial had ended. Only 25 percent of the participants were able to consume milk without symptoms. This was disappointing as, in the words of Dr. Robert Wood, director of pediatric allergy and immunology at Johns Hopkins: "Some of the more dramatic failures had looked like absolute successes in the study. They were tolerating huge amounts of milk; they were about as close to 'cured' as we could imagine."

Why would this be? Perhaps it was related to lifestyle. This was not discussed in the article. This article caused me to wonder if Rachel would remain allergy free in the long-term.

ALLERGIC ESOPHAGITIS
There was another troubling finding about oral immunotherapy. An article titled, "Relation between eosinophilic esophagitis and oral immunotherapy for

food allergy: a systematic review with meta-analysis"
noted that a new onset of EoE after OIT occurs in up
to 2.7% of patients with IgE-mediated food allergy undergoing this treatment strategy. According to Mayo
clinic, eosinophilic esophagitis is a buildup in the lining of the tube that connects your mouth to your stomach (esophagus). This buildup, which is a reaction to
foods, allergens or acid reflux, can inflame or injure
the esophageal tissue. Damaged esophageal tissue can
lead to difficulty swallowing or cause food to get caught
when you swallow.

This was a cause for concern. But there was no explanation of why these reactions were happening.

MAY 12, 2015: OIT TRIALS

I attended a local lecture with approximately 35
other people, titled "Food Allergy Research Update: Desensitization and Other Promising Treatments." It was
given by allergist Yamini Virkud, MD of Massachusetts
General Hospital. She spoke about current research on
food-specific immunotherapy and described a dozen or
so clinical Oral Immune Therapy trials being published
throughout the country and more ongoing. Each trial
consisted of a sample population of about 30 people,
with a success rate of 50-90% depending on how de-
fined they were and how they were analyzed.

Though she mentioned COFAR (Consortium of Food
Allergy Research), she did not make clear their role in
the process. I noted that there didn't appear to be one
overall larger organization managing the collective

findings of all this research, nor was there consistency in their methods or reporting.

She mentioned several patterns that had emerged with desensitization such as the failure of initial desensitization. Since it didn't work, this would cause twenty percent of study participants to drop out of the study and also cause GI or respiratory symptoms. She mentioned other patterns such as partial desensitization, complete desensitization, and complete tolerance. There were also many safety concerns with these studies because participants had reactions to approximately three percent of the OIT doses they were given.

I had wondered about the role of the mind-body connection in the findings. As the medical treatment or standard of care for food allergic patients was to avoid the foods they were allergic to and the patient's lifestyle revolved around this protocol, is it possible that failure could be attributed to the brain not having been retrained to accept this change prior to eating these foods. One cannot go from vigilant avoidance to stuff-your-face without retraining the brain!

The physician also spoke about all the ups and downs kids had as they went through the OIT treatments. The reactions sounded like they were worse than Rachel's processing.

The studies had similarities to Alexis's protocol. For instance, one study used probiotic and prebiotics to treat the gut. Yet there were some differences. For instance, another study used parasites, and a third used Chinese Medicine. None of the studies described Alexis's protocol of clearing the immune system or healing the gut prior to starting desensitization therapy or of using interventions to address the microbiome or mind/body connection.

This led me to wonder how much our success with the desensitization related to the protocol Alexis had devised. Of course, there's no way of knowing without research on the impact of using her techniques but I feel that intuitively this made sense. Another one of my philosophic mantras is: *Life is an experiment without a control group.*

In the meantime, the physician explained that the results of these OIT medical treatments were years away. Even if they showed favorable results, once the studies were concluded, physicians would still need to be trained in treatment methods.

Few allergists are going to try this procedure until there is a consensus for a standard protocol to follow that has proved safe and effective.

FECAL MICROBIOTA TRANSPLANTATION (FMT)

On May 18, 2016 I attended a lecture held by the Food Allergy Program hosted by The Division of Allergy and Immunology Research at Boston Children's Hospital. The most interesting and promising research that was presented during this lecture was that of Fecal Microbiota Transplanation. FMT was used in patients with C. difficile colitis (curative) and more recently with patients with peanut allergies. Among other study criteria measures, donors were trained to avoid peanut ingestion for one week prior to transplant. The study reported that 80% of people can get desensitized, and 20% of participants were desensitized during the 1st year. Closteria was needed in the probiotic to be effective.

This lecture was informative and confirmed for me the importance of a well-balanced microbiome for healing to occur.

Why do we need to do transplants when we can focus on healing our own microbiome? Learning new diet and lifestyle can help change this— proving an even greater need for health coaches.

WHEY PROTEIN
This article discusses the difference between first generation whey protein powders and modern concentrates. While the former contained as low as 30-40% protein and contained high amounts of lactose, fat, and undenatured proteins, the latter now contain as high as 70-80% plus protein with reduced amounts of lactose and fat. And they contain far higher levels of growth factors, such as IGF-1, TGF-1, and TGF-2, much higher levels of various phospholipids, and various bioactive lipids, such as conjugated linoleic acid (CLA), and often higher levels of immunoglobulins and lactoferrin.

Whey protein concentrates (WPCs) do have slightly less protein gram for gram than an isolate, and contain higher levels of fat (though these fats may in fact have beneficial effects) and higher levels of lactose but this should not give the impression that a well-made WPC is inherently inferior to a whey protein isolate (WPI) and may in fact be a superior choice, depending on the goals of the person.

According to 10 *Things the Processed Food Industry Doesn't Want You to Know,* "processing changes the way [foods] are digested and assimilated in your body." The article also states that "Processed foods contribute to an imbalanced inner ecosystem" and "Beneficial microflora cannot survive in your digestive tract when you are poisoning them."

There's also a difference between mechanical processing and chemical processing. Butter is a mechanically-processed food; the cream is separated from the milk and churned. When chemical processing occurs, all kinds of chemicals not necessarily listed on the label are used to provide things like texture, flavor, and color.

Appendix D
Food Comapnies Ditching Artificial Ingredients

Take Part wrote an article in June 2015 about *8 food companies that are ditching artificial ingredients.*

1. Papa John's—America's fourth-favorite pizza chain
2. Taco Bell
3. Kraft
4. Subway
5. General Mills
6. Nestle
7. Pizza Hut
8. McDonalds
9. Panera Bread

Even people without allergies should pay attention; we should all reduce the chemicals that we feed our bodies. The article mentioned the initial effort these companies are taking.

One more article of importance published by Vani Hari AKA The Food Babe on Dec. 29, 2016 summarized food companies who are eliminating toxins, antibiotics and GMO's from their products. Some of these companies include Campbells, Mars, Perdue, Kelloggs, and Del Monte.

We need to give these companies credit for acknowledging the issue, but we have a long way to go before our food supply and SAD (Standard American Diet) is considered "clean".

Appendix E
Recipes

Kugel Recipe from Camp: This recipe was given to me on an index card from one of the camp chefs during mother / daughter weekend. The kids loved this camp recipe, clearly because the ratio of sugar to all the other ingredients.

- 1lb pasta cooked – egg noodles
- 8 eggs
- 2 cups sugar
- 3 tablespoons Vanilla
- Apricot Jam
- Cinnamon

- Boil pasta.
- Beat together eggs, sugar, vanilla.
- Spread jam on bottom of pan.
- Add egg mixture to plain pasta.
- Place mixture in pan.
- Top with dollops of jam and sprinkle with cinnamon.
- Bake at 350° until set, about 25 minutes.

Recipe for Squash Souffle: (includes dairy and egg substitutes)
- 2 (10 oz.) pkgs. frozen butternut squash
- 1-1/2 sticks margarine
- 16 oz. non-dairy light soy product (soy based: usually found in the frozen section)
- 1 cup flour (wheat substitute: 1/2 cup potato starch and 1/2 cup oat or corn flour)
- 1 cup granulated sugar
- 6 eggs (egg substitute: EnerG egg replacer made from potato starch and tapioca flour and/or milled flax seed. I use both, each for 3 eggs.)
- 1-2 tsps. ground cinnamon

Substitutes:
- 1 tbsp milled flax seed + 3 tbsp water can replace 1 egg.
- 1 tbsp egg replacer + 1/4 cup warm water can replace 2 eggs.

Preheat oven to 350 degrees Fahrenheit. Grease a 9x13x2 inch baking pan. In a large bowl, beat the squash, margarine, non-dairy soy product, flour, sugar, and eggs (or substitutes) together and pour into prepared pan. Sprinkle top with cinnamon to taste and bake for 45 minutes or until set.

Recipe for Italian Wedding Soup:
- 1 Package Ground Chicken or Turkey
- ½ Cup Fregola Sarda Pasta or Barley

- 3 Ounces Baby Spinach
- 2 Cloves Garlic
- 1 Carrot
- 1 Parsnip
- 1 Yellow Onion
- 1 Stalk Celery
- 1 Bunch Parsley
- Seaweed (kelp cut into pices)
- 3 Tablespoons Chicken Demi-Glace
- Cup Grated Parmesan Cheese
- Cup Plain Breadcrumbs
- 1 Tablespoon Dulce flakes
- 1 Egg for meatballs (optional). If using, add some extra breadcrumbs

Note: You can use chicken broth and ¼ cup wine instead of adding demi-glace to water. Also, dulce flakes can always be substituted for salt and pepper.

- Chop the spinach. Mince the garlic, dice the onion, carrot, parsnip and celery. Pick the parsley leaves off the stems and mince the garlic.

- In a medium bowl, combine the package of ground meat, (egg), breadcrumbs, ¼ of the onion, half the garlic, dulse flakes, half the parmesan cheese and half the parsley (roughly chopping the leaves just before adding). Stir to thoroughly combine. Using your hands, form the mixture into 24 to 28 meatballs, each about 1 inch in diameter.

- In a medium pot, heat 2 teaspoons of olive oil on medium until hot. Add the carrot, celery, parsnip, ¾ of the onion and ½ of the garlic. Stir occasionally, 3 to 4 minutes, or until softened.

- To the pot of celery, carrots, etc, add the barley or pasta, demi-glace and 3 cups of water; season with salt and pepper or dulce flakes. Heat to boiling on high. Once boiling, add the meatballs and seaweed. Reduce the heat to medium-high and simmer, stirring occasionally, 5 to 6 minutes, or until the meatballs are cooked through. (You can test the doneness of your meatballs by remov-ing one from the pot and cutting it in half.)

- Once the meatballs are cooked through, stir the spinach into the pot of soup; season with salt and pepper to taste. Reduce the heat to medium-low and simmer 2 to 3 minutes, or until the spinach has completely wilted. Remove from heat.

- Serve and top your bowl with the rest of the parmesan cheese and parsley.

— *Recipe adapted from Blue Apron*

Resources

Food Allergy Research

Allergies and Your Gut. http://allergiesandyourgut. com/

Boyce, Joshua. "Guidelines for the Diagnosis and Management of Food Allergy in the United States." Journal of Allergy and Clinical Immu nology. https://www.ncbi.nlm.nih.gov/pmc/arti cles/PMC4241964/

Campbell-McBride, Natasha. Gut and Psychology Syndrome. Medinform Publishing, 2010.

Du Toit, George. "Randomized Trial of Peanut Con sumption in Infants at Risk for Peanut Allergy." New England Journal of Medicine. http://www. nejm.org/doi/full/10.1056/NEJMoa1414850

Food Allergy Research and Education (FARE). https://www.foodallergy.org/

Guidelines for the Diagnosis and Management of Food Allergy in the United States: *Report of the NIAID-Sponsored Expert Panel The Journal of Allergy and Clinical Immunology.* www.jacion line.org

Jackson, Kristen D. "Trends in Allergic Conditions Among Children: United States, 1997-2011." May 2013. NCHS Data Brief. https://www.cdc gov/nchs/data/databriefs/db121.pdf

Kilgour, Lisa. "How Your Digestion Controls Your Immune System" Collective Evolution. March 6, 2015. http://www.collective-evolution. com/2015/03/06/how-your-digestion-controls-your-immune system/

NAET: Nambudripad's Allergy Elimination Tech niques. https://www.naet.com/.

Pistener, Michael and Jennifer LeBovidge, "Living Confidently with Food Allergy." http://www. allergyhome.org/handbook/

Sandford, Kia. "The Truth About Frozen Yogurt and Ice Cream." https://www.aol.com/video/ view/the-truth-about-frozen-yogurt-and-ice-cream/554c574be4b07729e362d0bb/

Thernstrom, Melanie. "Allergy Buster: Can A Radi cal New Treatment Save Children with Severe Food Allergies?" The New York Times Maga zine. http://www.nytimes.com/2013/03/10/mag azine/can-a-radical-new-treatment-save-children-with-severe-allergies.html

Yong, Ed. I Contain Multitudes: The Microbes Within Us and a Grander View of Life. Ecco, 2016. http://www.newyorker.com/tech/elements/ breast-feeding-the-microbiome

Consortium of Food Allergy Research http://www.cofargroup.org/

http://onpoint.wbur.org/2015/02/26/ peanut-allergies-solutions-immunology

Resources for Allergic Kids

Food Allergy and Anaphylaxis Network, Alexander the Elephant Who Couldn't Eat Peanuts. Time Frame Productions, 1994.

Immune Tolerance Network, "Leap." http://www.leapstudy.co.uk/."Kids with Food Allergies." http://www.kidswithfoodallergies.org

Kingma, Theresa. Dairy-Free, Egg-Free, Kid Pleasing Recipes & Tips. Self published, 2004.

Health Coach Resources

The Institute for Integrative Nutrition. http://www.integrativenutrition.com/

Lipman, Dr. Frank. "The Be Well Blog." https://www.bewell.com/blog/

https://www.bewell.com/blog/allergy-treatment-probably-dont-know /

Your Food Allergy Coach http://www.yourfoodallergycoach.com/wp/blog/

https://www.ncbi.nlm.nih.gov/pubmed/25216976

https://www.allergychoices.com/about-the-la-crosse-method-practice-protocol/food-allergy-treatment /

http://www.pbs.org/wgbh/nova/next/body/your-microbiome-as-a-baby-may-influence-your-intestinal-health-today/

http://fitness.mercola.com/sites/fitness/archive/2011/05/11/whey-protein-shown-superior-to-other-milk-proteins-for-building-muscle.aspx

The Fecal Transplant: Can It Help Colitis, Candida, IBS and More? https://draxe.com/fecal-transplant/?utm_source=newsletter&utm_medium=email&utm_campaign=newsletter

The Tapping Solution http://www.thetappingsolution.com/what-is-eft-tapping/

How to do EFT tapping http://www.emofree.com/eft-tutorial/tapping-basics/how-to-do-eft.html

The Whey It Is: The Truth About Whey Protein! July 22, 2016. http://www.bodybuilding.com/content/the-whey-it-is-the-truth-about-whey-protein.html

https://authoritynutrition.com/9-ways-that-processed-foods-are-killing-people/

http://www.takepart.com/article/2015/06/30/8-food-companies-are-phasing-out-artificial-ingredients?cmpid=foodinc-fb

http://foodbabe.com/2016/12/29/my-favorite-moments-from-2016-see-which-food-companies-are-dropping-the-toxins/

Review From an Allergy Free Kid

After two years of lovingly and meticulously writing, re-writing and editing this manuscript, I forwarded a copy to Rachel, my eighth grade voracious reader for her review. She read some then looked up and said "Mom, it's really good. Honest! But these are your issues. I'm over it."

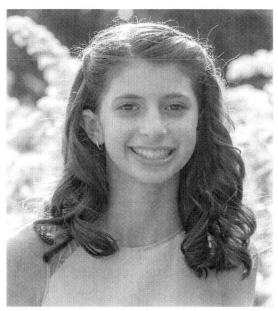

Gotta love that kid!

CPSIA information can be obtained
at www.ICGtesting.com
Printed in the USA
LVOW10s2208181217
560207LV00044B/2882/P